Fitness for the Unfit

Fitness for the Unfit

Ina Marx

A Citadel Press Book
Published by Carol Publishing Group

First Carol Publishing Group edition 1991

A Citadel Press Book
Published by Carol Publishing Group
Citadel Press is a registered trademark of
Carol Communications, Inc.

Editorial Offices   Sales & Distribution Offices
600 Madison Avenue   120 Enterprise Avenue
New York, NY 10022   Secaucus, NJ 07094

In Canada: Musson Book Company
A division of General Publishing Co. Limited
Don Mills, Ontario M3B 2T6

Photography by Jay Daniel
Design by John Goodchild at Triad
Originally published as *You Are in Charge*

Manufactured in the United States of America
10 9 8 7 6 5 4 3 2 1

Carol Publishing Group books are available at special discounts
for bulk purchases, for sales promotions, fund raising, or
educational purposes. Special editions can also be created to
specifications. For details contact: Special Sales Department,
Carol Publishing Group, 120 Enterprise Ave., Secaucus, NJ 07094

ISBN 0-8065-1264-4

To all my fellow travellers

Contents

Fitness for the Unfit

Introduction

"Know first that no urge, no influence, is greater than the will of the self to do what it determines to accomplish in any direction— whether physically, mentally, or spiritually." —Edgar Cayce

Yes, this is a "how-to-book," but not just another one of those self-help manuals to be read, shelved and forgotten.

It is intended to benefit everyone, of every sex and every age, but it may be of utmost importance to the victims of today's fitness scene. I appeal to the out-of-shape, out-of-breath, less than perfect average American who finds it impossible to live up to the standards and demands set by our present health and body conscious society. I extend a particular invitation as well as empathy to the many who feel old, think old and have allowed themselves to be programmed as "over the hill." To all of you who made the effort to compete, failed and threw in the towel, and those of you who never tried at all—let me show you the way to a new beginning! This book will encourage the disillusioned, the disheartened, the disabled and all the fitness dropouts to start anew. There is no doubt in my mind that the ideas I present will work for you and lead you to a better life—one of perfect bodily health, a sound mind and inner peace.

You have my personal guarantee. I will give you all the proof that you need in order to trust me as your authority, teacher and role-model. I will present you with the facts from my research and the details of my own experiences. This information can be corroborated by all those who have come to me and have been helped.

I will take you by the hand, if you let me, and lead you step by step to better health. I will provide you with a flexible practice routine as well as a follow-up plan. In fact, I will assist you as long as you need me. You may call this a training program instead of a book, because it is based on the teachings, classes, seminars and workshops that I have conducted over the past twenty years. My plan, which I call the IM Method, is not to be confused with work-outs, instant routines and miraculous overnight changes. Yes, it does require homework, dedication and commitment. But there is no grading and no one ever fails this course. Another chance is always available. There is no monetary output other than the purchase of this book. Nor is there a club to join, classes to sign up for or equipment to buy. The program is not complicated to follow and the book is easy to read. The commitment is to yourself only.

You are the only one who can be responsible for any change you desire. Responsibility goes hand in hand with adulthood or maturity, and means that you yourself are in charge of your life. You are the only one who can determine your life course. I would very much like to help you rid yourself of defeatist cliches, such as "I could never do that," "What will happen to me?" "I can never make up my mind," and especially "What will people think?" I urge you to understand that the societal standards that you try to live up to are, in fact, created and set by yourself. Maturity or wisdom is the right to make your own decisions without depending on the advice or approval of others.

As we learn to rely on ourselves, we bolster our self-confidence, which is perhaps the most important prerequisite for a meaningful existence. Self-confidence is gained by accomplishing that which we thought was impossible. That assurance evolves into self-love, the profoundest love of all, because you can't do what is best for you until you truly love yourself.

Self-confidence and self-love are the two steps that can lead to self-realization and the awakening of our spiritual nature. We can also keep going, if we so desire, until we arrive at complete enlightenment. We may not reach it in this lifetime, but it feels good to try.

This book will present you with the option to find freedom from outside influences. It can lead you to the liberation of the "you"—the most important person in the world. It is imperative to realize that you are unique and like no one else. You differ in age, height, bone structure and musculature from the next person. Your metabolism, genes and nervous system, chemical composition and tolerance are unequaled. The same exercise, foods and environmental conditioning that seem beneficial to someone else, may neither please you nor agree with you. For instance, today's fitness methods seem to be geared to the young, lithe and apparently indestructible body. Instead of saying: "This is not for me!" and retreating into your old rut, you can discover the fitness and general achievement level that works best for you. Rather than blindly following the latest fitness trends, diet programs, mind expansion fads, and emulating the "experts," you can learn to investigate your own potential and choose whatever suits your individual requirements.

I can tell you from my own experience that it feels terrific to be liberated from having to fit in and please others. Instead, I am able to please myself, convinced that there are no limitations to what I can achieve. Best of all is the knowledge that I no longer need to worry, be afraid or feel guilty.

How did I arrive at this exalted state? Well, it wasn't easy, nor did it happen quickly. But let me assure you that once you make the commitment to be in charge of your life, it gets easier with each step.

My own uphill climb began at age forty, which the average American considers the time to begin skidding downhill. I was totally devoid of self-confidence. Self-love and self-realization were not in my dictionary. I was indoctrinated from earliest childhood to believe that I was fat, lazy, stupid, defiant — that I would end up being nothing but a disgrace to those who sacrificed themselves for me. I do not blame the ones who were in charge of me then, because they did not know any better and acted in accordance with the standards of the ethnic background of their generation. I, in turn, *chose* to accept their predictions and struggled along with my limited capacities for most of my life, plodding through the motions of living as best I could. My life seemed to be a never-ending series of personal tragedies, which almost ended drastically when I was thirty.

At that time, I worked in one of the luxury resorts in the Catskill Mountains on weekends, while my husband stayed in New York City and took care of our little daughter. I received my salary along with board and a room in a ramshackle firetrap reserved for the hotel's help. I was pregnant again as well. One winter night, as the staff members were sleeping, fire broke out. I was in a room on the third floor, where many of us were trapped as spreading flames consumed the wooden staircase, cutting off our escape.

What saved me in the fire were my immediate instincts. The only possible way to escape was through the window. There were two in this third-floor dormitory. One was always stuck and the other was blocked by a crowd of the other panic-stricken occupants. I smashed the stuck window. When the flames came unbearably close I jumped, plummeting down onto a concrete drive. By the time the fire truck arrived, the building had burned to the ground and ten people were dead.

I survived. But I had fractured my back and pelvis, sustained internal injuries, cracked ribs, and broken my psyche as well. And I lost my unborn baby. I was first placed in a body cast. Later I graduated from a brace to a steel corset which I was told to wear for the rest of my life. Because I was in constant pain, I became addicted to tranquilizers, barbiturates, painkillers, and three packs of cigarettes a day. I suffered from fatigue, insomnia, and obesity. I spent all my time seeking relief from a succession of physicians and physical therapists, but no one could help me. I regarded myself as the innocent victim of circumstances. Life held no meaning for me, and I often contemplated suicide.

After two unsuccessful suicide attempts, psychiatric treatment was advised. I got better and somehow managed to function. I looked for work, but took on jobs I couldn't handle. I went to school and quit, joined organizations that bored me and attempted physical fitness programs that left me frustrated and in tears. My only successful venture during this period was the birth of our second daughter, but soon after I broke down again.

Innately I was a fighter. I found a new therapist and my mental attitude improved. Physically I was still a wreck, but I decided to hang in there and try every healing method that was suggested to me. None did me any good, but I refused to be discouraged.

One day someone advised, "Try Yoga!" I had never heard of Yoga, but latched onto it as a last resort and it worked miraculously for me. At first, my situation seemed hopeless. I could not bend in any direction. I had, however, found a sympathetic teacher. I was determined to stick to the instructions because I had caught a glimpse of a more hopeful future.

Discipline and hard work were the keys. In the past, I had always worked belligerently. Now I exerted a slow, steady deliberation, motivated by my purpose. I knew that consistency was the vital factor. I didn't turn my whole life over to Yoga, for I still had my family to take care of, but I practiced conscientiously for at least an hour each day. Sheer mechanical repetition brought everything together. My back grew stronger. After three months, I threw away my corset. My figure improved. I was healthier and more energetic. For the first

time in years I fell asleep easily. I gradually eliminated the tranquilizers and barbituates that had been a staple in my diet.
Quite naturally and painlessly I gave up smoking.

As my body changed, so did my mental outlook. Neither
drastic nor sudden, a different character manifested itself. My
sense of values changed as well as my attitude toward people. I
developed more patience, kindness and tolerance. A whole
new world of learning opened up to me. I found now that I
could teach Yoga and pass on the benefits that I had received
to as many people as I could teach. At age forty, I realized that
I, myself, am responsible for my state of being and that I can
attain any goal I desire.

At this writing, I am past sixty. According to medical and
societal standards, I am old. If I applied for a life insurance
policy or a job, I would undoubtedly be rejected. Since I no
longer subscribe to others' judgment, I maintain that age is
irrelevant. For me, life truly began at forty. I feel younger, healthier, and better looking than I did in my twenties. I am stronger and I have more energy, vitality, and optimism. I feel great
all the time and never get sick. I was chubby as a child and
thought to be "dumpy" as an adult. When I first began to practice Yoga, I was an out-of-proportion size sixteen. I changed
my figure to fit a well-proportioned size eight, and I retain that
shape to this day. I have become calm and peaceful. I came to
love myself and have learned to give love and to receive it. I
must still confront personal crises, but the more I grow spiritually, the easier they are to cope with.

While I do not follow the popular expectations for aging,
I do not yearn for youth. I feel sorry for those who cannot
accept growing older and are racing desperately to recapture
lost youth. There is no way to escape forever the exterior signs
of aging. Old age, however, is a state of mind that can be
changed. If your life has a purpose toward which you keep
striving, you can never grow old mentally or spiritually. Your
mind and body will not deteriorate if you keep them in peak
condition. The ravages of old age make headway only if an
organism is stagnant.

I genuinely look forward to each day and feel that there
are many good years ahead of me, that I have time to accomplish what I have yet to do in this lifetime. I refuse to be
defeated by the laws of probability and have defied the medical
diagnosis, "You must learn to live with your pain." I have dis-
proved the orthopedist's prescription which would have con-

fined me to a wheelchair for life. Although my back injuries have knitted, subsequent examinations have shown the deterioration of several discs and a congenital curvature of my spine. Those who view my x-rays find it incomprehensible that I can even walk. Yet my back is incredibly strong, supple, and free from pain.

Many people ask me, "How did you overcome all the odds against you? What is your secret?" It was really very simple, and it isn't a secret. To the stranger who inquires, "How can I get to Carnegie Hall?" the New Yorker answers, "Practice, practice, practice!" Practice is the key to my success. Success can come with any endeavor, from baking a perfect cake to winning a Nobel Prize — whatever pursuit fits an individual's inclinations. For me, it lies in physical accomplishment. My success is due to the consistency of my practice. I do not practice compulsively, but I do work out routinely, just as I brush my teeth or take a shower daily. Since it is in my nature to take chances, I may, at times, push myself too far, straining a muscle or tendon. At one time that would have caused me to panic and run for help. Now I have learned to ease the aggravation, let the pain subside by itself, and resume my routine slowly and sensibly.

Everyday practice requires self-discipline, but should not be rigid or compulsive. Self-discipline is one of the major requirements for a purposeful life. Discipline can be imposed, nonetheless, only if it is backed up by motivation. I think of motivation as choice. I believe that we all have the right to choose the direction in which we want to travel. Each one of us is blessed with free will. We can live this life in whatever way we see fit. We can opt either for progress and growth or procrastination and the *status quo*. We, ourselves, are the only ones able to judge ourselves and to aim for either success or failure. After years of being sad and sick, I chose to become happy and healthy. The choice was *mine*.

If you also wish to change and grow and transform, to enjoy life to its fullest, let me be your guide. I will lead you to optimal fitness and happiness. The direct way to bliss, Nirvana — or whatever else you desire — does not lie in intellectual musings or philosophical ponderings. It can be found in practical techniques which you can apply without outside help: physical exercise, correct breathing, proper nutrition, relaxation and meditation — in that order. This is the holistic route of integrating body, mind and spirit that works for everybody.

I hear objections: "How can physical exercise take precedence over meditation?" you want to know. "Why all the emphasis on the body? Is it not the mind that leads us on the spiritual path?" These are excellent points. A perfect body—totally fit and healthy—has little meaning if its owner's thought structure is faulty. On the other hand, those with severe handicaps who have a healthy attitude can overcome most of their obstacles and function profoundly.

The easiest way to effect a change of mind and gain control of thoughts is through the body, because the body is the more obliging of the two. It may also resist you at first, but the body is much less stubborn than the mind, especially if it is presented with the right incentive. Your physical anatomy will respond very quickly if you feed and exercise it properly, become aware of its functions, and respect it as an ingeniously, marvelously constructed instrument. Once we honestly tune in and listen to what it has to tell us, we can experience harmony with nature.

Detoxifying the body of all poisonous substances and purifying it through deep, powerful breathing clarifies our thoughts and increases our ability to concentrate. As we cleanse our body systems to eliminate the residue of harmful foods and chemicals and replace those with proper nutrients, we can expect to feel lighter and more wholesome. When the body becomes healthy and pure, we can then develop the higher aspects of mind and spirit and reach a state of transformation which surpasses our wildest dreams. Our thoughts will change naturally—all by themselves—toward optimism and peace. Slowly, we find ourselves gravitating toward meditation and other spiritual practices to reach the highest powers of our being. It happened to me. All I wanted was a strong back. As I started to move my body in the right direction, all the other bonuses fell into place.

I wrote one book when I was over forty, and another one when I reached my fifties. I promised to keep you posted on my progress at sixty and seventy-plus, and said that I planned to stand on my head at eighty and have a ball. It looks like I am going to keep that promise!

Part One
Physical Fitness

CHAPTER ONE

The IM Method
for Perfect Health

*I*M is the method I developed to achieve perfect health. It is tailored to the individual and designed for all people who haven't been able to successfully establish a fitness-oriented lifestyle for themselves. IM are my initials and they also stand for I AM or YOU ARE — the most important person in this world. You are like no one else, and only *you* can determine what is best for you. I have developed and perfected the IM Method during my twenty years of teaching many people in all walks of life, devoting myself to each individual as a unique being. The method is based on extensive research and my own experiences and growth. I could present you with volumes of testimony from my former students describing the beneficial results of my teachings. I chose, however, to present myself as the role model to demonstrate the rewards awaiting those who follow this program. While it may be geared to a certain audience of underachievers, it can be practiced by anyone from eight to eighty, regardless of physical condition. It is beneficial for the sports enthusiast and also for the very fit and flexible person. It is, without a doubt, extremely rewarding for those who are the overweight, underactive, sedentary majority of Americans. Everyone benefits from the IM Method to their individual degree of capability.

All the routines and postures shown in the picture section of the book are demonstrated in the beginning as well as intermediate versions. No one is held back and no one needs to compete. The techniques are derived from ancient Yogic practices, which have been adapted and custom tailored to suit the needs of our present hectic society. Yet, the IM Method is not a Yoga program per se, but a combination of practical routines which will fit into everyone's time schedule. The IM Method differs considerably from all other programs in today's fitness

scene. It does not advocate rigid routines or disciplines, needs
no mechanical devices or supervision by a "fitness expert." It is
not a sporadic "workout" or "build-up" or placid exercise for
the senior citizen. It neither promises you fast results nor
instant gratification. It guarantees, however, that obvious
benefits will come about pleasurably, without force, strain or
exhaustion. Anyone who practices the method will report
favorable changes, such as feeling better, looking better,
becoming younger and healthier. You can experience more
energy and vitality, eliminate colds, fatigue or insomnia, and
see back pains and other joint problems disappear. Being firm,
flexible and fit will become a way of life. Perhaps the greatest
benefits and changes will be felt on our non-physical or metaphysical levels, and these changes will manifest subtly and
effortlessly. The IM Method consists of static stretchings and
movements of the body, designed to condition every part of
the physique and the inner organs as well. Each exercise is
coordinated with the breath. Emphasis is on proper breathing
techniques—expertly taught. Practiced, they will become a
way of life and can prove to be a cure and prevention for physical and mental disease. Meditation and relaxation methods
comprise a major part of the regimen. Routinely performed,
they will impart secular as well as esoteric value to everyone.
Counseling on good nutrition and health habits are also part
of the curriculum. The IM Method is, in fact, a combination of
practical routines that coincide with yoga and other ancient
philosophies as well as with current holistic teachings.

What is the meaning of Holism or Wholism? It can be
spelled without the "W", but it represents the word "whole."
This is defined in the dictionary as: Containing all the parts
necessary to make up a total, undivided and undiminished;
entire; complete.

There is nothing new about Holism—it is an ancient concept with a new name. The Vedic writings of about 5000 B.C.
refer to man as part of the universe in body, mind and spirit.
All major religions, at one time, regarded man as part of a unity
or trinity. Most of the holistic practices, called "New Age," are
the "Old Age" ways of healing which the advancements of
medical science and technology obliterated. Herbology was
practiced in China in 3000 B.C., and acupuncture
and other oriental healing methods can be traced back even
further. Evidence suggests that the native American Indian
knew of natural cures for most diseases. Chiropractic and vari-

ous methods of massage and manipulation were practiced in this country at the beginning of the century.

We discarded our natural practices of healing when we entered the age of medical monopoly and turned into a sickness-oriented society. We became dependent on the world of medicine, the AMA and "our doctor." It was in "His" power to make us well, and he could do no wrong. We would unhesitatingly ingest and inject every medication, antibiotic and vaccine that he prescribed. We wanted instant relief and the doctor complied. We would undergo surgery at the drop of a hat, not daring to ask a second opinion.

But within the last decade we have discovered that the indiscriminate dispensing of drugs can be dangerous, even lethal. We have realized that too often surgeries are performed that are crippling, deadly and avoidable. We can no longer view medicine as always compassionate or the medical profession as having only an ethical interest in preserving life. Reimbursement policies have so changed that medical treatment is now dictated most of the time by government insurance programs and regulations. There are those persons, of course, perhaps still the majority in this country, who continue unhesitatingly to follow doctor's orders. They docilely fill their prescriptions, submit to triple bypasses, or undergo radiation or chemotherapy without seeking alternatives. But many others have discovered Holistic Health practices or Alternative Healing methods as the answer to their problems — to effect the cures that the medical profession has failed to provide. A good number of MD's, as well, have chosen to experiment in or to specialize in holistic practices. We now have holistic orthopedists, osteopaths, dentists and oculists in addition to the standard holistic or alternative healers in the field of acupuncture, acupressure, iridology, chiropractic, homeopathy, to name but a few. All holistic healers have this in common: They do not conform to allopathic medicine or treatment with drugs, and don't dispense synthetic supplements. They generally do not condone drastic methods of intervention through surgery or radiation. They maintain that effective treatment considers the whole organism and discovers the root of the problem, instead of isolating parts of the body and treating symptoms. They acknowledge the physical, mental, emotional and spiritual nature of each being. This is contrary to our present system of orthodox medicine, which is structured to separate and segmentize body and mind.

THE IM METHOD FOR PERFECT HEALTH

While today's practice of psychiatry is still regarded as the preferred non-medicinal form of treatment for mental and emotional illness, holistic methods and techniques have come to play a major role in the field of mental health. Many present-day therapists, including MD psychiatrists, are integrating guided imagery, meditation, relaxation, visualization and other unorthodox practices into their treatments. More realistic schools of psychotherapy, such as bio-energetics, gestalt therapy, primal therapy, or psychodrama, have replaced many traditional approaches.

Mind improvement, mind expansion and consciousness raising activities are flourishing. Our stress and strain society is frantically searching for relief from tension, mental illness and the mind/body separation. In response, the holistic movement provides a slew of behavioral modalities to choose from.

I believe that the leaders and practitioners in the holistic movement are basically sincere in their desire to help mankind. I would certainly consult or avail myself of holistic services if I had physical problems, before swallowing powerful medications or submitting to surgery. I would seek a holistic counselor for problems of the mind rather than undergoing long-term psychotherapy or becoming dependent on tranquilizers or other mind-altering chemicals.

Yet, while the holistic movement deplores separation of body, mind and spirit, they are causing fragmentation by the very multitude of methods that they employ. Each one is lauded as the real one, the only one that can help. As they focus on their specific systems of manipulations, nutritional therapies or centering techniques, they examine only one aspect of the whole, and are therefore subject to limitations. Holistic and alternative healing methods are undoubtedly valuable to our present society and certainly less dangerous in their application than most medical treatments. But I personally feel that everyone needs to work in conjunction with all other holistic methods for holism to be truly comprehensive and effective. The same holds true for modern medicine, psychiatry and other health regimens.

Medicine and psychiatry will not truly help us achieve mental and physical health until they abandon all fractionalized and symptomatic treatment and consider the whole person's physical and psychological make-up. Medicine is making headway in acknowledging the body-mind connection. Ulcers, colitis and asthma are no longer the only diseases thought to be psychosomatic or psychogenic. It is conceded that arthritis, diabetes and other familiar and socially accepted ailments may also be of mental origin, as well as the major killer—cardiovascular disease. Conversely, millions of dollars are still spent looking for cancer cures in the laboratory—instead of investigating prevention in the mind. If we can assume that some diseases originate in the mind, is it not logical to suppose that almost all diseases are the result of destructive thinking?

Psychiatry in general still tends to overlook the body as the cause for numerous mental illnesses despite the mounting scientific evidence that many psychoses have a physiological base. Many people, who are actually suffering from physical dysfunctions, such as hypoglycemia or other chemical imbalances, are still diagnosed as psychotics or schizophrenics.

Real progress in health care can only occur when medical, psychiatric as well as holistic practices come to view each person as a unique individual whose parts affect, reflect and compliment the whole. It may sound utopian, but it is possible to foresee that one day all healers will acknowledge each other and work together for the betterment for the human race.

But where do we stand at present and where do we go from here? We can first of all realize that good health is our birthright. We are all born whole. Even those with mental and physical imperfections possess the potential for wellness. We are created as a self-contained unit of natural resources and our system is designed to avoid sickness and fight illness—if we use it properly. We have existed and survived through the stone and ice ages, withstanding their dangers. We were able to live in wilderness and remote regions of this earth and be entirely self-sufficient. Today there exist tribes and civilizations, in isolated areas in the Himalayas, Nepal, Mongolia and other places of the world that are totally independent in their health maintenance and sickness prevention, living better, fuller and much longer lives than we in the midst of sophisticated science and technology. Yet, we too, as "civilized" human beings, can be in charge of our health if we comprehend the correlation of body, mind and spirit and learn to rely on our inherent powers for survival. We don't have to hold outside forces, beyond our jurisdiction, responsible for our ills and ails. We can stop blaming background, genes, germs, viruses and bacteria, pollution and weather conditions for our poor state of health. We can also face the fact that we cannot abuse, neglect or hurt our physical and emotional systems and get

THE IM METHOD FOR PERFECT HEALTH

away with it. If we don't exercise, live entirely on junk food, and deliberately subject our bodies to cigarette smoke, alcohol, drugs, and harmful chemicals—we cannot expect to stay healthy. Excessive destructive thinking will also lead to our mental and spiritual deterioration. Holistic philosophy maintains that attitude is the sole factor in creating our state of mental, physical and spiritual health, that it is our thought system instead of outside conditions and circumstances that determines the quality and course of our lives.

Generally, we do not need to be sick—but sometimes we are. And that is natural, because animals get sick, and so do plants and trees. Yin and Yang, positive and negative poles, action and reaction are the balancing forces in human existence. Dis-ease is nature's way of letting us know that we need to rebalance our systems. And since we are not as self-sufficient and united with nature as the Yogi who lives in the high mountains of India, we do need healers. It is imperative that we exercise common sense and choose appropriate treatment at those times that we require the assistance of the healing profession. It makes sense to consult a chiropractor when we have a whiplash injury or to turn to acupuncture for relief of migraines and painful arthritis. But it would be downright foolish to refuse antibiotics or resist surgery if we had an acute infection or burst appendix. The right medication given at the right time to the right person can work wonders, and surgical procedures, when indicated, can save lives. Everyone and everything can be helpful—the physician, psychiatrist, holistic healer—the shaman and the spiritual guru. All methods, systems and ideologies work if they are applied in the right way. There is truth in everything, but no method or treatment is a panacea. There is no ultimate authority and nobody has all the answers. Someone or something can lead you on the way, but no one can be with you all the time, and ultimately you yourself have to take over.

The IM Method will show you the way, not to autonomy, but to the liberation of your self. Through its practice you will discover that you are not just a body, but also a mind and a spirit. As you become aware of your body by exercising it correctly and learn to know its anatomy, the body will let you know if something is amiss or out of whack. Once you understand how to tune into your body and listen to what it has to say, you will be able to control its functions. When you oxygenate your system, cleanse your organs through deep breathing, provide your insides with proper food and elimination, you experience health and harmony. When you are truly in touch with your body through deep relaxation, you will make a natural transition into the realms of your mind. Meditation practice will come about easily, without force, strain or effort, and the exploration into the spiritual aspects of your true nature will gradually evolve.

As much as anything can be a panacea or a cure-all, I am sure that the IM Method fits the bill. I am the living proof that it works. At one time I was the sickest person alive, but today I am well all the time.

The IM Method will teach you that you alone are responsible for your state of well-being, and make you aware that you can change whatever you want without fear. Most importantly, it provides you with all the tools needed to achieve good health as well as happiness and peace. The following practice guide will make your job easy.

Your Everyday Practice Guide

I will now give you a choice of methods and techniques to help you achieve greater health, and explain their functions and benefits in full detail. It is up to you to adapt them to your individual needs, incorporate them into your lifestyle, and practice them on a daily basis. Yes, it's daily practice which is essential to your progress—actually any progress, in any field of endeavor. Anything worth achieving and holding onto requires diligent and most often purely mechanical practice. A person may be born with a natural talent for singing, dancing, or painting, but unless he works to develop that talent, it will amount to nothing. The daily repetition of scales, pliés, or brush strokes is necessary to make a successful artist, and it is the consistency of the practice that brings the desired results. The same holds true for this course of personal integration that you are undertaking.

I trust that you have discovered by now that all methods work if you apply them. It is not the method but the self-discipline of everyday practice that will produce success. I am sure that in the past you have embarked on exercise, diet or mind-improvement courses, mostly because they promised you fast results and overnight miracles. You may have entered into them with great enthusiasm and even experienced beneficial results. Yet when the course ended, you fell right back into your old, destructive patterns. Or else you enrolled in a self-

help program which a) somebody talked you into, b) everybody was doing, and c) you paid good money for and were
determined to try "even if it kills me!" So you gave yourself a
push and a shove and coerced yourself into action. You may
have joined a health club and worked the machines and
pumped the iron, or invested in an exercising gadget of your
own. Or you attended aerobic classes, exercised in front of the
television, jogged or ran and joined TM, EST, or other consciousness raising activities. You felt better, looked better,
became trimmer, firmer and more peaceful.

But then came the inevitable day when your enthusiasm
began to ebb, then disappeared completely. You just couldn't
stand the thought of another weight lift, jog in the snow, ride
on the exercycle or repetition of the mantra. If you think that
your case is unique, be assured it's not. For instance, glance at
the Sunday newspapers listing pages of used exercise equipment for sale, sometimes to be had just for the hauling.

Don't berate yourself for lack of willpower, for most physical and mental self-improvement plans are doomed to failure.
No sporadic, haphazard, part-time or quickie program has
ever worked in the long run. And no one is going to voluntarily keep doing something he or she doesn't like. Furthermore,
when you have to force yourself into performance because it
may be good for you, you are definitely defeating your purpose. All the tensions that you bring to a task you dislike are
harmful to your body and psyche.

The key to lifelong fitness is to establish a program that
fits into your everyday schedule. It must be uncomplicated,
take a minimum of time and require no gadgets, special equipment, instructor or manipulator at your side. It must be fun to
do, and it must bring progressively evident results.

The IM Method is designed to meet all these requirements. You will experience obvious improvements in a relatively short time. It is not just a combination of exercise, diet
and meditation, and it is definitely not a "work-out." It is a way
to restructure your life! You will look forward to your daily
practice and once you have established it as part of your daily
routine, it will become a part of you and you won't want to
give it up. If you skip the exercises, your system will let you
know that it is missing something vital for its well-being. Yes,
this course requires self-discipline. I purposely use the term
"self-discipline" instead of willpower, because willpower
implies forcing yourself to do something against your nature,

whereas self-discipline means simply fulfilling an obligation to yourself. You do have to be prepared to work toward your achievement. In the beginning you may have to give yourself that little push to set aside the time for practice, especially when you think you are too busy, too tired or too unmotivated to keep it up. After a short time the momentum of the program will take over; you'll find that you no longer need to push, for the routines will have become part of you.

Here are some *don'ts* to remember as you start:

Don't confuse push with rush. Don't start with the idea of accomplishing as much as you possibly can in the shortest span of time. The eager beaver who wants to do everything immediately and throws himself into a frenzy of practice, never sticks to any regimen very long and is forever rushing into something new.

Don't become impatient with your body if at first it seems resistant to your wishes. The back that won't straighten or the knees that won't bend will respond sooner and better to gentle prodding than to brute force. The same holds true for your mind, which will want to wander as soon as you sit down to meditate.

Don't set your goals too high, especially in the beginning. Be aware of your present capacity and accept it. While you should not decide that certain techniques are impossible for you to perform, don't strive for perfection just yet. Concentrate on improving each action to the best of your ability. When you can say, "I can't do this now, but someday I will," you have grasped the meaning of self-improvement and are well on the way to success.

Don't ever become frantic about your practice. While you should practice consistently, don't feel guilty if you have to skip a day either due to circumstances, or just because you feel like goofing off.

Don't set any goals for practice or achievement. The only goal required now is your awareness.

The following are suggestions for how to structure and facilitate your daily practice plan:

When to Practice

It is helpful to stick to a regular practice time and adhere to it as much as possible. The morning is best of all, as you will start off your day vibrant—with your body, mind and emotions alert and ready. The physical practice is a little more difficult in the morning, in that the body contracts during sleep and is generally more stiff than in the evening. A warm shower or bath to loosen up will definitely help. I would recommend this practice time for any working person. It will enable you to move through the day with added calmness, concentration and energy. If you feel that you are too tired or too busy at this time, train yourself to get up earlier. Your loss of sleep will be compensated by bursts of vitality and alertness.

Those who stay at home, especially homemakers, whose early morning hours are taken up by preparing breakfast and getting the family off to school or to work, may find the hour before lunch or in the late afternoon a good time to practice.

Some people prefer evening practice to relax them after their day. Others whose evenings are taken up find that their preferred time is the hour before going to bed. Such a routine will undoubtedly induce a sound and restful sleep.

How to Practice

Empty Stomach: One reason that early morning practice is preferable, is that the stomach is really empty. You should never practice on a full stomach. No exercise and no sport should be performed immediately after a meal. This is not only for the sake of comfort, but a physiological necessity, because exercise causes a compression of your organs that can interfere with your digestive and excretory systems. Breathing practices, relaxation and meditation techniques, as well, become uncomfortable, and a sense of fullness interferes with your ability to concentrate. Try to wait three hours after a meal, and two hours after a snack before you begin to practice.

Location: Try to choose a place that is conducive to performing your routines in a leisurely way. Ideally (and this means under ideal weather conditions and surroundings), one should practice out-of-doors, especially meditation. Otherwise, try to find a space that is quiet, well ventilated, and carpeted, if possible. It need not be spacious, as the only equipment you require is a towel and possibly a small pillow to sit on as you meditate. The freer your practice time is from distractions, such as children and dogs and telephones, the better will be the results. A full-length mirror is very helpful as you exercise.

Dress: The choice of dress (or undress) is purely a matter of preference. The only requirement is that there be no restriction of movement, no binding, belts, or pressure from elastics. Shorts are fine, so are bathing suits or leotards. Keep all body distractions out—no hair that has to be adjusted or pushed from the eyes, no jewelry to get in the way, etc.

Length of Practice

Physical Exercise: I suggest that you start by devoting twenty minutes a day to exercise. Eventually you may want to practice longer, maybe as much as an hour. I am aware that other fitness and work-out programs you took in the past may have lasted much longer, perhaps one to two hours. But did you do them on a daily basis? Please believe me when I impress upon you that it is not the time length but the consistency of practice that brings the desired results. Even ten minutes of steady exercise per day will keep you in optimal fitness, more than one or two hours of practice every other day. Follow the exercise plan that I have outlined for you in the pictorial section. Here are some general hints:

Do not be upset if you do not understand all the details of the directions for the postures. As you practice with growing awareness, you will understand more and more. The pictures are of completed postures. You are to go only as far as you can and use the pictures for direction. Concentrate on working both sides of the body evenly and moving slowly and gracefully.

Most likely, you are beginning with a body that is out of condition. Therefore, regard your body as unused territory that will need patient cultivation. You will be setting to work joints, muscles, tendons, and ligaments that have long lain dormant. Be gentle, and don't expect the impossible right away. You will have to condition your body slowly by stretching muscles and loosening joints that until now have had little or no exercise at all.

Eventually you will reach your goal of firmness and flexibility, but straining and jerking your body won't get you there. Don't worry about reaching the ultimate position in the beginning. Your body will benefit from even the partial execution or hold of the exercise. Even when you think you're not getting anywhere, your body will be stretching a little at a time. Provide your body with the incentive and it will do the rest.

Perform your favorite aerobic activities or sports, such as accelerated walking, hiking, bicycling or swimming on a regular basis. Aim for three times per week—at the least.

Breathing: Allow yourself at least ten to fifteen minutes of structured breathing practice twice a day in the beginning. Try to do the breathing either before or after the other exercises.

Choose a comfortable sitting position in the same undisturbed atmosphere. Concentrate on the Alternate Nostril and Bellows Breath as regular daily routines. Practice the other breathing techniques, either sitting or lying down, until you have mastered them. Then try to incorporate them into your daily activities until they become your everyday good habits. Practice the Glottis Breath in conjunction with the postures.

Complete Relaxation: I recommend that you end your practice session with the Complete Relaxation. You can also do it any time you feel tense or fatigued or sleepless. Always lie flat on the floor on your back, eyes closed, your whole body relaxed. Cover yourself with a light blanket when chilled. Follow the relaxation routine as described on page 87.

Meditation: Successful meditation is not measured by time. Even five minutes of daily practice is extremely beneficial. Start with five minutes the first week, ten minutes the second, fifteen minutes the third, and build up to twenty minutes of blissful silence. Like the other disciplines, meditation requires everyday practice. It is the steady routine that produces all the benefits. Meditation can be done anywhere, but it is most effective when performed in pleasant surroundings. But wherever or whenever you meditate, be sure to choose a quiet place and a time that you will not be interrupted. You need to sit with your back, neck and head in one line either crosslegged on the floor or on a chair with a straight back. You could also combine your breathing with the meditation; the Alternate Nostril Breathing especially will help to lull you into a very receptive state of mind.

You can meditate anytime. Early morning, of course, is best, but any time of the day or evening that suits your schedule and needs is fine.

CHAPTER TWO

What is Physical Fitness?

Fitness has become such a national obsession that it is nearly impossible to be unaware of the benefits of physical fitness to good health: increased energy and stamina, weight reduction, improved mental attitude, even an extended life. Americans initiated this crusade in the 1970s, and today fitness is an integral part of our lifestyle. It is advocated and endorsed by educators, physicians and politicians; it is almost un-American not to be engaged in some kind of exercise or sport.

In the not-so-distant past, we thought of physical activity as playing ball with the kids, golfing on Sunday, or engaging in an occasional game of tennis. Serious athletic events were something we watched on television, cheering our favorite team, drinking beer and munching snacks. Those who did attend exercise classes were often considered eccentric. But faced with the grim statistics of how inactivity can cause obesity, health problems and premature death, we changed our ways. We did this almost overnight, as is our custom as single-minded enthusiasts. In the process, we plunged from abject sedentarism into frenzied activity, ignoring the ill effects of such an extreme change.

After more than a decade of dedication to strenuous exercise, we are now told by authorities to slow down. The injuries and permanent disabilities caused by the fitness mania are too prevalent and serious to be ignored. Because of jogging and running, our knees, shins, Achilles tendons, feet and lower backs have suffered. We have sustained fractures, ruptures, strains, sprains and tears. These have affected all parts of our anatomy: bones, muscles, joints, tendons and ligaments. Excessive aerobic activity—dancing, bouncing and jumping— is reported to be the cause of stress and injury especially to the female musculo-skeletal system. It is common knowledge that heavy work-outs and marathon running for women can interfere with the menstrual cycle, causing eventual bone loss and osteoporosis in later years. Passé are those who expound, "You can never exercise too hard" or "There is no gain without pain." Exercise classes have been modified and aerobics routines have been renamed low-stress, non-impact, controlled or nonballistic. The very same fitness figures who spurred us on in the first place are now cautioning against the hazards of over-exercising. The newest books to flood the market deal with injury prevention. Jogging, running and aerobic work-outs are still around, but there is a damper on our enthusiasm. Many are running scared.

Something went wrong with the fitness movement. We began with the best intentions — to be healthy and fit. But because we expect instant gratification — instant food, instant medicine, instant bliss — we wanted it yesterday. We did not take enough time to prepare for training, to evaluate our potential, to check the credentials of those who called themselves experts, teachers and coaches. We rushed headlong into every new program because we didn't want to be left out. Allowing ourselves to be side-tracked from our original goal of fitness, we became obsessed with our physical image.

Big, bulging muscles were thought to be the epitome of a perfect male physique. Women, too, "pumped iron" to sculpt their figures or to spot reduce. Flab was a four-letter word. We combatted it with tummy tucks, fanny firmers and inner-thigh toners. But we missed the boat by neglecting the major requirement for optimal health and fitness: flexibility. We did stretch, but we did it impatiently, improperly, and we stretched the wrong muscles.

The most significant area for structural suppleness is in the lower back or lumbar, and its flexibility depends on the hamstrings, the large set of tendons in the back of the knee. Nearly all the stretching connected with running and aerobics classes centered on the calves and thighs, foreshortening and tensing the hamstrings themselves. That excessive bumping, pounding and stomping placed extreme pressure on the lower back, which should have been counteracted by slow, static forward bends. With the exception of professional gymnastics, modern dance and some of the martial arts, our present exercise systems have contributed to a decrease in spinal flexibility. We used to be able to touch our toes. Now we can hardly touch our knees.

My personal measuring rod of total health and fitness is the ability to bend forward, touching the head to the knees without bending them, and placing the hands flat on the floor, without pain. If a person of eighty can do this, I will guarantee without any further testing that he or she is in perfect health, cardiovascular or otherwise. A strong, healthy heart is a most valuable asset. Yet while accelerated or aerobic activity is vital to increased heart performance, this is not an indication of overall health. The heart is a muscle, but only one in a system of more than 600 in our body. With all the emphasis on strengthening the heart, we have ignored the importance of the rest of our musculature.

Today's jogger can probably increase his longevity, but it may not be fun to be old and suffer from tendonitis, injured kneecaps, or various spinal injuries. Preoccupied with the fear of a heart attack, we forget that the spine is our lifeline. Structural disorders are more prevalent than cardiovascular and related ailments in the United States. We are besieged by degenerative, chronic diseases such as bursitis, sciatica, spondelytis, arthritis, osteoporosis, along with sacroiliac and vertebral disc problems. Chronic back, knee and joint dysfunctions along with the standard "lower back pain" can lead to mental disturbance and depression, interfering with sexual and social enjoyments. We blame genetic and hereditary influences or organic diseases as the cause. Or we claim stress is responsible for our structural diseases, poor posture and proneness to injuries, as well as other ills and problems. We fail to examine the way our misguided fitness mania may have contributed to our chronic aliments, especially as we get older.

The physical conditioning we provide for our children is also greatly insufficient. Exercise programs in other parts of the world are often superior to ours and usually begin with pre-school youngsters. America's physical education programs are limited to game playing in kindergarten, coordination builders in elementary school, and in high school primarily preparation for sports: push-ups, sit-ups and jumping jacks. Fitness in college is geared to sports performance and competition. Everyone seems to be training for a spectator event, directing his energies toward Olympic achievement. The promotion of the athlete is a national industry, bringing in high profits to big business and the media. While the prestigious athlete may earn an enormous salary, he is more likely to suffer from physical mishaps, especially if he pursues his sport single-mindedly without a balanced regimen.

American athletes in general are in poor physical condition. They are prone to strains, pulls, dislocated discs and vertebrae, structural fractures and chips. The physiological and psychological tensions produced by competitive performance increase the body's vulnerability to accidents. Many depend on steroids and other harmful drugs to see them through the game. Today, sports medicine is flourishing and necessary. Athletes are having problems with lower back suppleness which leads later to neck, shoulder and upper back tightening as well. Ball and racquet games demand extreme forward movement of the muscles without counteraction. In their teens, athletes have already shortened their hamstrings and the muscles in the back of the leg. Unless athletes learn to tune and develop the rest of their structure as part of their training, it seems inevitable they will eventually suffer from structural disease. Not only the professional, but today's amateur athlete competing in marathons, biathlons, or triathlons is subjecting his body to punishment. Every human structure that is whipped, driven and tortured into performance will eventually rebel.

Sensible exercise, however, is a must for everyone. Unlike the automobile, the human body does not wear out with use. In fact, it is more likely to deteriorate from lack of use. The older one gets, the more necessary it is to keep up rather than decrease the body's activity. Performed correctly, exercise is not tiring because it increases energy which, in turn, creates more energy. But to avoid injuries, it is essential to be aware of the mechanics of physical fitness and the way these mechanics work in your own body. Instead of being swayed by what others say, learn to pay attention to your own feelings. Listen to the advice of your inherent common sense to determine what is right for you.

Exercise Choices

Basic requirements for maximum overall fitness are aerobics, flexibility, strength, balance coordination and relaxation. To date, no single program in today's fitness scene has been tailored to address all of these components. Sports alone do not provide you with complete physical exercise. The only way to condition the entire body and obtain overall fitness is through a system correctly called exercise: a program of bilateral, rhythmic movement which incorporates flexion, extension and rotation of the entire body. To give you lasting results, exercise must be done consistently, preferably every day.

Regular exercising is the most significant factor in attaining, maintaining and restoring health and vigor. A realistic system will prolong your life and make the difference between feeling tired and old, and feeling full of energy and great. Exercise is essential for everyone, no matter what your age or condition.

The overweight avoid activity with the excuse that exercising will increase their appetite. Nothing could be less true. Sporadic activity may make you hungry, but steady exercise acts as a stabilizer. Regular exercise reduces the desire for large quantities of food. While you may lose weight by dieting and counting calories, it is impossible to retain the weight loss without systematic workouts. Reducing by dietary methods alone, sacrifices the lean muscle tissue that is needed by the body. Exercise helps you lose fat and tone muscle. Without it, your muscle turns to flab, making you weak, tired and discouraged, ultimately motivating you to return to old, fattening eating habits. Body weight cannot be lost by exercising alone, but you can lose inches by doing nothing but exercising. Once the body is rhythmically activated, it is able to handle food in the most efficient manner. Exercise also acts as an aid to digestion, because it helps the body process and assimilate foodstuffs.

Everyone can do some kind of exercise that is good for them. Elderly individuals who are given the incentive and opportunity will benefit enormously, both physically and mentally, from mild activity. Even those in wheelchairs can be taught to use their upper bodies. Many paraplegics and amputees have achieved amazing feats through consistent training and sheer dedication. They participate in wheelchair marathon running and ski racing with the aid of ropes. Some have organized ball teams and their own Olympic competitions.

Many of us are less than perfectly constructed, with some defect, disabling tendency or sensitivity. These can be minor structural, neurological or organic limitations. If you have been active in a sport since childhood, you may safely continue into old age, because the body has adapted to those particular patterns of movement. On the other hand, it is senseless to begin strenuous pursuits in later years without considering existing problems or weaknesses. If you have fallen arches, varicose veins or an inflexible lower back, entering suddenly into such vigorous pastimes as running, tennis or racquetball will cause you pain and possible damage.

Amateur running is rewarding and exhilarating if carried out in a nonpunishing form such as windsprinting, which incorporates graceful, rhythmic strides, good balance and coordination. Be aware that not everyone's physique is constructed for running. I personally feel that *no one's* body is designed for jogging, and that it is an unnatural form of movement. Hitting concrete with short, bouncing steps, aptly called jogs, jolts the inner organs and can cause painful muscular and skeletal damage. Not even the most expensive athletic shoe is going to prevent a harmful degree of impact, especially if you run on asphalt.

Two alternatives to running and jogging are the rebounder and various forms of walking. A rebounder is a small trampoline which is quite inexpensive (far less than a health club membership). With the rebounder you can run, jog and bounce to your heart's content, achieving the same aerobic and euphoric benefits in a minimum of time. You will not be pounding your body into an unyielding surface, and you're not limited by weather conditions. Regardless of physical limitations (or just being shy about jumping in public), you will never hurt yourself.

Brisk walking is an excellent activity, and race or health walking is definitely superior to jogging and offers the same cardiovascular benefits as jogging. It has been popular in Europe for a long time, and was introduced as an Olympic sport in 1906. It is fast gaining acclaim in this country as well, because it is more energizing and revitalizing, and less strenuous than jogging and carries no risk of injury. Race walking also provides exercise for the entire body. Not only the legs, but hips, waist, the entire back, and shoulders and arms are involved in the movement. It can be practiced by everyone of every age. Men and women in their seventies and eighties are entering race-walking competitions. One enticing bonus, especially for females, is the prospect of becoming slim, trim, firm, and tight. Excess fat in the back of the upper arms, back of thighs, belly and gluteus maximus can actually be eradicated. I can personally attest to this. I am a dedicated race walker, and I consider the activity to be a pleasurable, healthful and aerobic adjunct to my exercise program. Race walking is, however, not all that easy to learn. If you wish to execute it correctly and eventually participate in racing, you will need instructions. In major cities, you'll find instructions available at public parks and recreation centers, generally free of charge. You may have to do some inquiring and phoning, but I can promise you that it is worth your while.

If you have played singles tennis, skated or skied all your life, you have nothing to worry about. But if you begin a sport in middle age, be wise and proceed with caution until you build up your flexibility and stamina. Cycling is one of the finest aerobic exercises for stimulating the cardiovascular system. A stationary bicycle gives you the same benefits as outdoor biking, but is not nearly as much fun! To those who cannot cycle, walk, walk, walk! You cannot overdo it. Because of inadequate transit facilities, New Yorkers have discovered walking, sub-stituting sneakers for high-heeled shoes on the way to the office. As a result, overweight Manhattanites are a rare breed.

Hiking is a great activity for leisure time, excellent for aerobic conditioning, overall strength, stamina and general exhilaration. It prolongs youthfulness, benefiting young and old alike. There are quite a few Manhattan executives who have discovered forests, rugged terrain or mountainous areas near the city. They spend at least one day a week, all year round, on a ten-to-fifteen mile fitness hike. This activity enables them to release tensions in body and mind, so their perfor-mance in the business world is improved.

Swimming is a splendid sport — a natural and perfect exer-cise as well as a relaxing leisure activity. It definitely keeps you young. Vigorous swimming not only builds arm, shoulder and leg muscles, but also provides a quality of aerobic exertion that equals jogging. Swimming alleviates and often cures many back, shoulder and knee ailments. The crawl and butterfly stroke are excellent for conditioned swimmers, but the gentler breast stroke and back stroke are better suited to precarious anatomies. Today, water exercises are practiced in most pool areas. They can be performed vigorously to strengthen and firm muscles and induce general body energy. Therapeutically, they are of considerable value as rehabilitative techniques. They are certainly harmless and can be fun as well.

For those near the mountains who can get away during the winter, cross-country skiing is a fabulous over-all exercise, using almost every muscle in the body. It does require training and special equipment, but it is much less dangerous and com-plicated than downhill skiing. Both young and old experience invigoration, increase in strength and performance level, plus a profound sense of well-being.

If running and jogging make you feel good, if aerobic

workouts to rock music are fun for you, and working with weights and gym equipment makes your day — pursue these activities by all means. If you are into rock climbing, wind surfing, hang gliding or similar feats — more power to you! But please bear in mind that none of the above-mentioned activities can provide you with overall fitness. You need to combine them with a routine of appropriate stretches in order to remain flexible and injury free.

Dancing is a wonderful recreation and excellent exercise for keeping you young and happy. Jazz, modern and ballet are usually appropriate for the young and energetic, but ballroom, folk, square and disco dancing can be enjoyed at any age. Of great popularity are the martial arts imported from the East. Judo, jiujitsu, karate, aikido or kung-fu are practiced as feats of strength and generally promote great physical fitness, agility and endurance. Most of them, however, require a degree of good physical condition and are best suited to young people. T'ai Chi Chuan can be practiced by everyone. It is gentle, nonstrenuous and pleasant to perform, but it does require instruction by a trained teacher, especially for the Westerner.

Keep in mind that your body thrives on constant motion. There is always a way to add pleasurable movement to your lifestyle. Excessive sitting, driving and lying down deteriorate rather than relax your body. Even if you hold a sedentary nine-to-five job and lack money or time for a health club, you can always devise ways to keep yourself moving. And those who adhere to a steady exercise schedule can increase their fitness potential with these additional practices:

1. Substitute walking for driving or riding whenever possible; it usually takes longer to wait for the bus than to walk.

2. Try to develop a brisk rather than ambling stride. It makes all the difference in aerobic activity.

3. Don't waste time waiting for elevators. Climbing stairs provides wonderful aerobic conditioning. It also strengthens every part of the leg.

4. Manipulate your body whenever possible: when you get up, before you retire, in your office chair, talking on the telephone. Use breaks at work to stretch, twist and bend, instead of dashing for the coffee machine. If performed correctly, all necessary chores like housework, weeding the garden, shoveling snow and washing the car can also serve as part of your fitness program.

CHAPTER THREE

Demystifying Yoga

Any activity is preferable to inertia, and all forms of exercise and movement are valuable to good health. However, for maximum conditioning all the muscles in the body must be attended to.

One system of exercise that reaches every part of the musculo-skeletal system and exercises the inner organs as well as the outer body is Hatha Yoga, the physical aspect of Yoga. Yoga exercises are patterned after the natural movement of animals. They are executed slowly, gracefully and thoughtfully. Forcing and straining do not have any place in this regimen. In many of our favorite fast-moving exercises, the muscles are bunched, jerked, and thereby foreshortened. Using these methods trains them to snap back like rubber bands. Yoga slowly stretches and elongates the muscles, elasticizing them in the process and increasing their resistance to fat deposits. This system allows you to acquire flexibility, increasing vitality, energy and stamina. At the same time, your inner organs and skeletal structure are conditioned. This therapeutic activity can retard the aging process and prevent deterioration of the bones. It provides relief from back ailments and improves or eliminates most diseases. In some form, Yoga can be practiced at any age by every person. The movements and postures can be adapted for every individual structure and body type. Movements range from simple stretches in the beginning to extremely acrobatic maneuvers for those who desire the challenge.

Cosmetically, this system goes far beyond spot-reducing. It allows you to retone, reshape, and recondition the entire body, distributing the inches in all the right places. Flab, sags, bulges and wrinkles can be prevented or alleviated. The most significant aspect of Yoga, however, is that all exercises are accompanied by regulated breathing. While we take the act of breathing for granted, it is more essential to life than anything else. We can live without food and drink for certain periods of time, but we perish if we are deprived of breath for even a few moments.

Most physical educators and medical authorities have long ignored the importance of correct breathing to good health. Only opera singers and other performing artists, it seems, have been singled out for instruction in proper breathing. Today the situation is changing and the healthful power of breath is becoming more widely recognized. People with acute respiratory illnesses, natural childbirth practitioners, and quite a few psychiatric patients are now taught Yoga breathing. Sport educators and some physicians realize the necessity for special breath patterns in conjunction with exercise, although much of their instruction is incomplete, focusing on shallow, open-mouth panting. It seems strange that it should be necessary to teach something as natural as breathing, especially since we are born breathing correctly, exercising our full lung power. But as we were either bottle-fed or pacified, our supply of air may have been diminished. Being swaddled in blankets as infants also may have restricted our movements and suppressed our natural air flow.

Yoga trains us to breathe slowly and deeply from the diaphragm, using the total capacity of our lungs and purifying the ingested air by inhaling only through the nose. This method permits a greater amount of oxygen to reach the heart (benefiting the entire cardiovascular system) and the brain (increasing mental alertness and clarity of thought). As deep, rhythmic breathing becomes a way of life, our system is purged of toxic materials from the environment.

To the novice, the long list of benefits to be derived from Yoga may seem unbelievable. I can personally vouch for all the benefits through both my own experiences and those of my students and other practitioners of Yoga I have known. These benefits have been corroborated by both medical and holistic professionals during my twenty years of teaching.

Yoga exercises, especially the abdominal ones, promote normalization and stimulate healthy functioning of the liver, spleen, kidneys and all the organs of the digestive system without medication or laxatives. They can alleviate indigestion, constipation, heartburn, chronic gastritis and colitis.

The inverted positions have multiple effects benefiting many parts of the body. They help to rest and strengthen the heart. They enable blood to flow freely into the organs and glands situated in the upper body, where the heart normally has to pump against gravity. The increased circulation to the thyroid gland stimulates its proper functioning in regulating the body's metabolism. This is an important factor in weight control and general vitality. The increased blood supply to the brain also helps to dispel fatigue and promote mental alertness. In the Shoulderstand, especially, pressure is removed from the blood vessels in the legs, minimizing swelling and painful symptoms of varicose veins. Menstrual cramps can be relieved and menstrual periods normalized.

The back-bending positions, as well, aid menstrual irregularities and can also be sexually rejuvenating to men and women. Stimulation of the gonads can correct the physical causes of impotence, frigidity and other sexual inadequacies. It can also strengthen the kidneys and favorably affect the urinary system.

Following a routine of overall Yoga exercises can most definitely help arthritic conditions. Arthritis cripples millions of people in this country, but no prevention or cure has been found as yet. The drugs that are offered to arthritis sufferers may partially relieve the symptoms but cannot cure the disease. Arthritis victims and sufferers from other rheumatoid diseases whom I have worked with have experienced a new lease on life from practicing Yoga. The exercises relieve stiffness and pain in their joints. It does, of course, require great courage and patience and initial pain to manipulate joints that are inflamed, and some persons may choose to revert to drug therapy. Those who do persist will discover that the gentle, gradual stretchings of Yoga can alleviate arthritis and other inflammatory conditions.

All Yoga exercises are particularly well adapted to the relief and avoidance of chronic degenerative diseases. Abuse of the body plays a major role in contracting the diseases, but physical inactivity is equally at fault for vulnerability to heart disease, arteriosclerosis, degenerative disc disease and osteoporosis. The latter, especially, is a major medical concern for post-menopausal women, and operations for hip replacements are perhaps the most common surgical procedures in our present society. The best program for preventing complications of osteoporosis in both men and women is a steady routine of Yoga exercising. Such a practice stimulates bones to retain calcium as they bear weight as muscles pull on them in various poses. A calcium-rich diet, of course, is effective as well. Other skeletal deteriorations and perhaps all structural diseases and imbalances respond to Yoga positions and movements. Yoga has been designed to promote complete flexibility of the entire musculoskeletal system, regardless of existing symptoms and injuries. My own success is just one case of many.

When it comes to the aging process, Yoga cannot stop the clock, but it can slow it down. Old age does not have to be a time of feebleness, sickness and depression. Inactivity and the discouraged attitude that accompanies it accelerate the aging process. Proper exercise can decelerate and, in some cases, reverse the process by increasing vitality, restoring flexibility, promoting healthy functioning of the organs and glands, improving blood circulation, controlling weight and firming muscles. I have taught students in their seventies and eighties who had more physical vigor than people half their age. As a group, they suffered less from the ailments that are so common among old people, discomforts like constipation, muscular stiffness and low resistance to respiratory infections. It is, of course, much better to begin maintaining a healthy body with exercise in youth rather than old age. But it is never too late to start Yoga. Because Yoga exercises are nonstrenuous, older people can find a plan of exercise that won't cause undue fatigue.

Ten years ago Yoga enjoyed great popularity. While the medical profession never officially endorsed Yoga, quite a few physicians, particularly orthopedists, advised their patients to try Yoga exercises. Serious athletes incapacitated by sprains, pulls or tendonitis, discovered that using Yoga as a warm-up system could help correct existing conditions and strengthen weakened muscles. Professional coaches recognized that Yoga stretches, relaxation and breathing techniques could improve sports performance and prevent injuries if practiced prior to competition. European athletic teams still continue to use Yoga as part of their training. Yoga never stopped being popular in such sports-minded countries as Australia and New Zealand. and in Europe. Dedicated Yoga teachers and practitioners are still around in the U.S., but theirs is a low-profile existence at present.

There are several reasons for this. Certain popular television programs showed Indian Yogis performing incredible acts, twisting themselves into pretzel shapes or compacting their bodies into small crates. While their feats may have been admired as freakish marvels, they inspired few to try Yoga. Also, as aerobic exercises gained in popularity, Yoga fell from favor because of its reputation for slow, consistent movement that does not incite cardiovascular acceleration. Actually—when Yoga is carried out in its truest form with dynamic breathing, it can be as invigorating and powerful as any other aerobic workout. The average Yoga practitioner, however, will benefit from additional accelerated movement. I have always encouraged my students to combine their Yoga routines with various aerobic activities and/or sports for extra cardiovascular stimulation.

Another misconception about Yoga is that it is a religion rather than an exercise system. It is true that some followers, especially in India, treat Yoga as a religion, complete with rites, prayers and chanting. But Yoga is not a religion. It is a set of ethics, applicable to wholesome functioning in everyday life. Yoga exercises can be practiced without any involvement in rituals, nor do the exercises interfere with devotion to any religion.

The practice of Yoga does require discipline. So does every endeavor that is meaningful and of lasting value. Yoga is different from other sporadic exercises which are soon replaced or discarded. It is a progressive series of exercises, directed toward daily improvement, that leads to eventual perfection of the body. Practice is essential, but it need not be carried to an extreme. As little as fifteen minutes each day will produce obvious results in a short period of time.

Those who criticize Yoga will point out that some classic postures, the Shoulderstand, Plough and Bow, can be dangerous for people with certain neck and back problems. On the contrary, these particular postures (and all Yoga positions) were designed as a system of therapeutic practice to correct, strengthen and improve most structural afflictions. Each individual, however, must be considered unique. Every good Yoga teacher will pay special attention to those with specific problems, instructing them on modified positions in the beginning, then gradually working toward standard ones.

Classic Yoga is associated with headstands and sitting in the Lotus pose, but successful practice does not depend on performing these positions. While periodic inversion of the body is advocated for circulatory and cardiovascular benefits, many equally effective poses can be substituted for the Headstand. Sitting in the Lotus position and squatting require limber, flexible knee joints. These positions come easily to children, Hindus, and people who have been conditioned through cultural habits to sit in this fashion. But it is not a natural position for most adult Westerners. It would be foolish and dangerous for a teacher to demand a student to force his or her body into the Lotus.

Though it may not be a current fad, Yoga is still very much in evidence in exercise salons and health clubs, and athletic meets as well. But the new terms for it are stretching, posture improvement, or sports conditioning. Because everyone is aware of the importance of stretching, there are many books and classes on the topic. Yet most stretches are really Yoga postures. True Yoga is much more than simple stretching. Yoga positions incorporate a static stretch that is held much more steadily and for longer periods of time than other stretching exercises. Yoga stretches are designed to balance each side of the body for total physical harmony and release of tension. Emphasis is also directed to the slow, unbroken motion of entering and leaving each position as well as to the even flow of breath. Actually, any calisthenic, rhythmic or dance movement can become a Yoga pose by holding the body in a static position and accompanying this with proper breath control.

All methods of correctly devised exercise work if you apply them consistently. Self-discipline — the daily practice of what you have learned — is the only way to get desired results. Someone, some system or some publication can lead you on the way, but no one can be with you all the time, except yourself. Ultimately, you cannot attend classes for the rest of your life, and at some point you have to take over and maintain your own program. The key to lifetime fitness is to establish a routine that is feasible within your personal lifestyle. To complete it everyday, your selected program must be uncomplicated, take a minimum of time, and require no gadgets, special equipment or instructor. After each session, you should feel refreshed, relaxed and revitalized. Any physical activity that leaves you exhausted, drained or muscle-bound is defeating your purpose and should be discarded. The system that is individually designed for you must bring progressive results that you can see. Above all, it should be enjoyable. These two achievements will give you the incentive to be a regular practitioner.

CHAPTER FOUR

Your Breath is Your Life

P hilosophers, scholars and thinkers throughout history have acknowledged that the secret of life can be found in the function of the breath. The importance of the breath is mentioned in the Egyptian *Book of the Dead,* and in the ancient Chinese healing texts dating back to 2000 B.C. The Book of Genesis in the Bible states, "The Lord formed man of dust of the ground and breathed into his nostrils the breath of life, and man became a living soul." The Yogis discovered centuries ago that breathing is the elixir of life. They developed it into a veritable science as well as an art form that could be practically applied for every human need. The principles of Hatha Yoga outline instructions for the techniques of breathing.

Hatha is the Yoga of physical culture, combining body stretching postures and regulated breathing to produce the utmost flexibility, health and vitality. The word Hatha comes from the Sanskrit words "Ha" meaning the sun and "Tha" meaning the moon. It refers to the balance of these two forces, corresponding to the positive and negative forces in the body. Hatha Yoga teaches us that the flow of breath through the right nostril is controlled by the sun, through the left nostril by the moon, and that the proper balance of these breaths leads to the unification of body and mind and total harmony of all the systems.

The practice of Yogic techniques and breathing can lead us to the attainment of optimal physical and mental health. The combination of proper exercise and nutrition and controlled breathing is the prerequisite for a long, healthy and meaningful life. Those who want to travel further will find these healthful practices provide a base from which they can move from material existence toward spiritual growth and harmony with all things.

It is the rare person in our society who knows how to breathe properly and is conscious of the breath. Open-mouth breathing is taken for granted, and physical fitness authorities still consider good posture as "shoulders back, chest out, belly in." This posture is actually the antithesis to correct posture and inhibits correct breathing. Various physical education teachers and sports team coaches may slap you on the back and order you to "Breathe!" Well-meaning people will tell you to get out into the open air and "take a really deep breath." But once there you're left hanging, because no one has explained what to do with that breath and where to put it.

It is strange that it should be necessary to teach something as natural as breathing. Yet, chances are we would not be doing something as natural as walking upright if we were not taught how. A child raised by four-legged creatures would walk on all fours and not straighten his body. If we were brought up in a mute society, we would never learn how to speak. Some functions are intrinsic to us, others must be acquired. Correct breathing fits into both categories. We are born with the ability to breathe naturally and correctly, exercising our full lung capacity. If you observe a baby lying on its back, you can see his abdomen rising and contracting gently while the mouth is closed. This indicates that the breath flows naturally in and out of the nostrils. We forfeited our natural ability as we adopted unhealthful habits and environments. Restrictive garments, for adults as well as babies, have contributed to unnatural breathing. While today's woman is liberated from tight girdles and corsets, she is still cutting off her circulation with tight-fitting pants, skirts and bras, and men wear constricting belts and ties. Because we sit or stand for long hours with poor posture in air-conditioned or over-heated offices, our generally sedentary work helps to establish incorrect and inadequate respiration. The stresses and strains of our modern society and general ignorance of proper relaxation, contribute, as well as derive from, bad breathing habits.

Some people exist in high altitudes amidst pure air. The Hunzas, for example, live in the high, thin air of the Himalayas, and have developed their lungs fully to obtain necessary oxygen. They must use their entire lung capacity to breathe and are motivated to inhale through the nose. They are rarely affected by disease and have been proven to live longer than the average man. Like the Hunzas, Yogis and those who have been instructed in Yoga breathing know how to breathe correctly. Today's sports physicians, athletic coaches and fitness instructors realize the importance of conscious breathing, but most of their instructions focus on open-mouth breathing. There is little emphasis on the inhale and therefore the exhale has no meaning.

During active sports, the lungs do work to their full capacity, but unsystematically with spasmodic, jerky movements. The increased oxygen intake is immediately consumed as a result of the constant loss of energy. Most active sports and exercise performers end up exhausted and out of breath and are prone to injury and heart attacks. There is no rhythm in unconscious breathing, and the laws of nature dictate rhythmic movement: from the beating of the heart, to the vibration of the atom. Swimming is perhaps the only sport that induces rhythmic breathing and forces you to control your breathing. It is impossible to swim vigorously and engage in shallow breathing.

Treatment of certain ailments through proper breathing techniques is popular in many countries. Ayurvedic medicine has long been practiced in India, stressing diet, herbs, natural medication, Hatha Yoga and breathing exercises. Sanatoria in Switzerland long ago recognized the combination of high altitude and pure breathing as the most powerful method of curing tuberculosis. Fresh air and improved breathing methods are also among the chief measures now used in Russian health centers for regeneration and the continuance of good health into old age. China has established Breathing Clinics where the only form of treatment for various illnesses is rest and specified periods of deep breathing.

In the United States, many medical doctors have recognized the adjunctive benefits of proper breathing techniques for the treatment of asthma, bronchitis, emphysema, certain heart conditions and hypertension. Some dentists, psychotherapists, chiropractors, and all holistic health practitioners advise or instruct their patients to breathe deeply either during treatment or as a separate endeavor.

Unfortunately, very few professionals are experts on breathing. Even advocates of natural childbirth, whose methods center on the breath to release pain and facilitate birthing, are teaching breathing techniques that are basically incorrect. Correct breathing means to breathe air through the nose and exhale through the nose, whenever possible. Inhalation through the mouth (except when swimming and running) is not essentially beneficial to your health. Air taken in through the mouth is cold, dry and uncleansed as it enters the windpipe and brings with it the risk of infection and colds. The nose, however, possesses an ingenious filtering system enabling us to inhale air that is warm and pure. The combination of tiny hairs and mucous membranes in the nose strain out most of the impurities and toxins in the air, with the result that cleaner air is brought into the lungs. When we breathe out through the nostrils rather than the mouth, the lungs gain more stamina since they take longer to deflate.

The other important aspect of good breathing is to breathe from the diaphragm. Our everyday breathing habits are often just the opposite: we suck in the stomach as we inhale and release it as we exhale. We are then engaging in shallow breathing, partially inflating the lungs, using only the upper and middle lobes. We are using only a third of our lung capacity and rarely are the lower lobes either activated or oxygenated. Our lungs become flaccid and atrophied causing and abetting a lack of stamina, as well as a proneness to respiratory and other debilitating diseases.

In Yoga or other diaphragmatic breathing, we push out the abdomen as we breathe in, lowering the diaphragm and thereby providing the lungs with maximum space for expansion. With all this room to expand, the lungs completely inflate, like balloons, down to the very bottom. This rarely happens in our routine breathing. Generally we employ clavicular or thoracic or upper chest breathing, which raises only the ribs, shoulders and collar bone, and uses only the upper lobes of the lungs. Correct breathing is rhythmic, relaxed and above all, controlled. When you learn the simple, common sense mechanics of breathing, you can master, direct and apply the breath at will.

There are many benefits to proper breathing. Good healthy lung tissues resist bacteria. One is unlikely to catch colds, flus, or other viral diseases and will be resistant to infectious germs when lung tissue is strengthened. Sinusitis and other nasal inflammations, migraines and other headaches can be relieved by improved breathing.

Deep breathing affects the natural functioning of the internal organs. Liver, stomach, pancreas, and all abdominal organs are stimulated by the mild pressure exerted on the organs during diaphragmatic breathing. Regulated breathing promotes cardiopulmonary and cardiovascular efficiency by sending freshly oxygenated blood cells to the heart and through the entire body. Also, the workload of the entire cardiorespiratory system is reduced by 50 percent by changing from thoracic to diaphragmatic breathing.

Chronic bronchitis sufferers have great difficulty in breathing, aggravated by a distressing cough and general lack of resistance. Regulated breathing can control the coughing and breathlessness, even when acute inflammation is present. This is also true for emphysema, where shortness of breath is ever present, and coughing and fear of asphyxiation encourage shallow breathing, apprehension and tension. While the loss of elasticity in lung tissue cannot be restored, the practice of correct breathing techniques gives relief to the sufferer by reducing fear and nervous tension.

Asthmatics can be completely cured through a regimen of proper breathing exercises regardless of whether the origins of the asthma are nervous, emotional, allergic or infectious. Asthma is a prevalent disease in our culture and many children are affected. A bad asthma attack is a shattering experience, as the muscles controlling the bronchioles go into spasm. Air can get in but not out of the lungs, and the victim struggles for breath but is virtually breathless. Drugs prescribed for asthmatics have proven not only useless in controlling and preventing the attacks, but most of them, especially cortisone and its derivatives, have caused devastating side effects. Many doctors today are recommending Yoga breathing for asthmatics. Abdominal Breathing and relaxation techniques can combat the vicious circle of attacks and the fear and tension which precipitate them. With consistent practice of breathing techniques, the seizures can undoubtedly be eliminated.

There exists, of course, a fine line between physiological and psychological illnesses and sufferings, but whether or not the condition is psychosomatic or not is of no consequence to the relief or cure. It is important to realize, however, that the breath is the key mediating factor between the mind and the body. Insomnia, fatigue, lack of appetite, indigestion, or constipation may have a physical or emotional cause, but all of them can be helped by learning how to breathe in a slow, controlled manner.

The most common complaint in today's Western world is nervous tension and stress, which is one and the same. The prevalence of stress is evidenced by the enormous amount of tranquilizers, sedatives and drugs which are produced and ingested. The frustrations, challenges and competitiveness of our times lead to worry, anger, anxiety, fear and other destructive emotions which, when counteracted by palliatives, may cause emotional breakdowns and mental disorders.

Regulated breathing is one of the most effective methods to restore mental equilibrium and balance. As you practice the exercises you learn to relax, periodically relieving yourself of the mental tension before it builds up to its overflowing point. Fear tightens the stomach, anger raises the blood pressure, and anxiety brings on palpitations. Most of our diseases are the result of uncontrolled emotions. If you are angry, you can instantly calm yourself by consciously slowing down the breath and making sure not to hold it at any time. All emotional upsets and turmoils can subside and eventually disappear with consistent practice of breathing and relaxation exercises.

We can easily control pain with rhythmic breathing and often alleviate it: during labor and in childbirth, during the menstrual cycle when many women are prone to suffer, and when undergoing dental work. Slow, deep breathing will calm the nerves and soothe the system, and the mind can be turned away from the pain.

Energy and stamina can be increased through proper aeration of the entire system. Everyone possesses a storehouse of potential energy which is not released without conscious effort. Dynamic breathing releases this untapped energy, thereby vastly increasing one's endurance and vigor. When you feel tired and mentally fatigued, ten minutes of Bellows Breathing (refer to page 53) can act as a wonderful revitalizer.

The same exercises that provide extra energy can also promote sound sleep. Insomnia can be relieved and often cured with practice of the Complete Breath (page 51). Yogic breathing also ensures an increased supply of oxygen to the brain, thus improving mental alertness and clarity of thought. Any breathing method, especially the Alternate Nostril Technique (see page 52), practiced right before a school test or an audition, improves concentration and relieves anxiety at the same time.

Yoga breathing is an invaluable tool to counteract addictions. If you honestly decide to give up smoking, for instance, you can train your body and mind to want to stop smoking. When you begin the breathing exercises, you will be bringing more air into your lungs than you have known for years. As you begin to master the exercises, you will find your lungs clearing up, nasal congestion relieved and your throat free from dryness. With the increased supply of oxygen to the system, the desire to smoke can be eradicated. The forceful breathing of the Bellows Breath will get rid of the poisonous tobacco pollution that has settled on the walls of your lungs.

For the overeater, the urge to devour the forbidden piece of chocolate or ice cream can be suppressed by shifting the concentration to the breath. It is a powerful substitute for the craving and can help you not only lose weight, but keep it off. Breathing techniques with other relaxation techniques are part of the reeducation program in many Drug Rehabilitation Centers. Anyone who seriously wants to break the drug habit will find Yoga methods to be of enormous help.

Healthy skin is another benefit from deep breathing. Women spend millions of dollars annually on creams and lotions that promise beautiful, radiant complexions. They could save themselves much time, money and disappointment if they realized that what goes on top of the skin is less important than what is going on beneath it. The most effective cosmetic for a glowing, healthy-looking complexion is good circulation. Healthy circulation enriches skin tissue and eliminates poisons that cause skin eruptions. Yoga breathings are designed to stimulate circulation and purify the blood.

Deep breathing by both partners can also lead to an improved and more fulfilling sex life. This is aptly and graphically depicted in the many volumes on Tantra Yoga. Emphasis is on rhythmic breathing to calm and relax the lovers and sublimate the sexual energy so that orgasm is controlled and foreplay is enjoyed to the utmost. Yoga breathings both stimulate and balance the endocrine system and can reenergize and correct sluggishly functioning sex glands.

The spiritual or esoteric aspect of Yogic breathing is referred to as Pranayama. Ancient Eastern tradition holds that every individual is destined to draw a limited number of breaths during the course of his years on earth. If he can slow down the rate of his respiration, then he can postpone his death. Many Yogis and holy men practiced this restraint of breath and their longevity was phenomenal.

Pranayama is the conscious practice of controlling Prana through concentration and regulated breathing. Yama in Sanskrit means purification, and Prana means life force or life energy. The Chinese call it "Chi," the Japanese "Ki," and the Hebrew writings refer to it as "Ruach." Western scientists believe that the entire universe is filled with "ether," which also corresponds to Prana. Essential to life, Prana is found in every living thing from the most elementary form of plant life to the most complex form of animal life. It is in matter, but it is not matter. It is in the air, but it is not air. Too subtle to be graphically pinpointed, Prana exists as surely as do electricity and cosmic rays. Its abstract quality is comparable to that which is termed the soul. The soul is commonly accepted as a spiritual part of every individual, although it cannot be seen. In the same way, we can understand the existence of Prana. Perhaps the closest we can come to the concept of Prana is vitality. This special vitality reveals itself, to all those who seriously practice Yoga, as a definite element of our physical and mental constitution.

Prana is taken into the body with the breath in advanced Yoga breathing. Devout Yogis and those who strive toward enlightenment devote much of their time to concentration and meditation and to the mastering of the breath. These sages have surpassed the physical techniques of Yoga and are concerned with the mental methods that purify the mind, stimulate nervous centers, develop higher faculties and control the senses. This mental control is said to lead to psychic powers, and especially Samadhi (see page 127), the ultimate state of consciousness. Many Yogis employ extremely difficult and advanced breathing techniques. They are able to inhale and exhale at great lengths, lock or seal the breath in the nose or throat, and store the Prana in the vital centers of the autonomous nervous system. They can direct the breath to every organ and part of the body and hold it there for long periods. Their emphasis is on breath retention for the purpose of supreme control of all earthly function. Some Yogis can suspend their breaths indefinitely and have survived being buried alive for long periods. While we may not be striving toward Samadhi in this lifetime, the more simple breathing techniques, practiced regularly, can open the way to better health, serenity and a heightened spirit as well.

I am limiting the following instructions to the practices which are easy to perform and don't require the assistance of a skilled teacher. You need not spend much time at one sitting but they should be done routinely, with consistent practice, in order to bring success. Except for the Glottis Breathing, you practice the breathing exercises separately from the other exercises. If you get into the good habit of doing them just prior to your other exercises, you will feel the added advantage of having your body fully oxygenated and relaxed.

Remember that all breathing is done through the nose with the mouth closed, especially in the beginning of your practice. Never hold an inhale longer than you are ready to. It is better to take an extra breath. As you become more proficient, you will be better able to hold and eventually control your breathing at all times. This is your ultimate aim. Eventually, controlled breathing will become a natural habit. But don't concern yourself with it in the beginning. Everything will come together naturally with continued practice.

We are working toward the Complete Breath using the entire lung capacity. I have simplified the procedures by dividing the breath into three parts: abdominal, intercostal or rib cage, and clavicular. Practice these routines either lying on your back with your knees slightly bent, sitting on the floor, sitting on a chair, or standing up. Your back needs to be straight in all the breathing routines.

Abdominal Breath

Even though you are breathing from the diaphragm, make believe that the breath originates from the abdomen. Lightly place your hand on your abdomen and think of this area as a balloon which you will fill with each inhale and totally empty with each exhale. Breathe in slowly through the nose. Feel the expansion of the abdomen and the air filling your lungs as one unified process. You will feel your fingers spreading apart and your hands separating as your abdomen fills. Exhale slowly through your nose. The air coming out and the contraction of the abdomen are as one process. Repeat three times. Each time try to balloon out more with the inhale and push out more air with the exhale.

There are many opportunities outside your routine practice session to use this very simple but most essential breathing method: Lying in bed, riding in a car, sitting in a dentist's or other office, or standing in line in a supermarket. I encourage you to practice as often as possible. The technique is the opposite of the way that you have been breathing up to now, and the more you reinforce the new technique, the better. Eventually you will be able to empty yourself of wastes and toxins, and consequently take in much more fresh air.

Intercostal Breath

Place your hands on your rib cage. Start by having your thumbs right up under the breast with the heels of the hands on the sides of the rib cage, and the fingers pointing toward the front. Picture your rib cage as an accordion. Slowly inhale, expanding the ribs sideways. Feel the ribs separating from each other and the tissues spreading. Think of the muscle expansion and the breath as one integrated movement. Then slowly exhaling, let the ribs come together accordion fashion. Strive to expel all stale air, wastes and toxins. Repeat three times.

Clavicular Breath

Gently place your fingertips on the clavicular area above the chest. Inhale slowly. From the inside, feel the back of the throat fill with air. On the outside, feel your hands moving where they lie on your chest. Exhale slowly, emptying the lungs totally. Practice three times.

Complete Breath

Practice these first three breathings until you feel comfortable with them. Then you will be ready to combine the three elements of abdominal, intercostal and clavicular breaths into one smooth, flowing "complete breath."

It is now preferable to sit on the floor or in a chair, holding your back, head, and neck in a straight line. You may rest your hands on your knees or in your lap, but in the beginning it is advisable to rest the fingertips lightly on your abdomen to make sure that you are performing the exercise correctly. Empty your lungs before starting. To the count of eight, inhale deeply while pushing out your abdomen, rib cage and chest. Hold your breath in the back of your nose for eight slow counts. Start exhaling slowly to the count of eight, contracting your chest, rib cage and abdomen. Some people find it more comfortable to exhale and contract first the abdomen, then the rib cage, and last the clavicular region. This is a matter of personal preference and is also correct. When you have completed exhalation, your abdomen and the surrounding areas should be hollow. Relax the abdomen and pause ten seconds. Perform three times.

Try to gradually increase the length of inhalation and exhalation to twelve seconds, and the holding of the breath to the count of twenty. When you have comfortably reached this stage, slowly increase the period of holding your breath by five counts at a time. Remember, never strain to hold your breath longer than you can. The exhalation should always be controlled.

The various steps of the exercise should be performed in a continuous flowing movement. You can practice this breathing to fill out "dead time" during the day. It is also enormously helpful to remember as an immediate tranquilizer in moments of acute anxiety or pain.

Alternate Nostril Breath or Pranayama (preceding meditation)

This is also called sun and moon breathing. The right nostril takes in the sun breath and the left nostril the moon breath. Some teachers prescribe counting with this exercise but I find it distracting. Inhale and exhale as slowly as possible without counting. You can add the counting later if you want to, the ratio of one-three-two. For instance, inhale to the count of four, hold the breath for twelve counts, exhale eight.

Sit in a comfortable position with the spine erect. Extend the thumb and last two fingers of your right hand (if you are left-handed, use your left hand), bending down the middle and index fingers. You may need some practice with this but don't struggle. If it feels too uncomfortable, keep the middle and index finger extended. Close your right nostril with your right thumb and let all the stale air gush out of the left nostril. Now inhale deeply through the left nostril and close it with the last two extended fingers. Both nostrils are closed. Retain the breath for at least two seconds, eventually holding the breath for longer and longer periods without discomfort. Now remove the thumb and let the air flow out the right nostril with as much control as you can. Immediately inhale again through the right nostril, close off both nostrils, retain the breath for as long as you can, and then remove the two fingers over the left nostril and slowly exhale. This is one round.

In the beginning, practice two more rounds without removing the fingers from the nostrils. Gradually increase to six rounds. Eventually you will want to devote at least ten minutes of time to this practice.

The benefits of this particular technique are vast and its effects are astounding. You are learning to balance the opposite currents in your body. Alternate Nostril Breathing helps restore your equilibrium. In the beginning, you will inhale and exhale more easily on one side than the other because your nasal passages are not balanced and the air is drawn up unevenly. With practice, you can achieve an even and controlled flow of air through each nostril, resulting in improved physical balance. The breathing promotes calmness and serenity by affecting the balance of the nervous system as well. It relieves sinus conditions by helping to dissolve obstructions in the sinus cavity and facilitates unobstructed breathing by opening the nasal passages. Regular practice will prevent nasal colds, or you can use the technique at the onset of a cold or headache to head off any discomfort. This technique can also cure insomnia. As of Pranayama, the Alternate Nostril method prepares the body and mind for meditation, making you more receptive to stillness.

Charging or Bellows Breath

As you do this breathing exercise, picture your lungs as a bellows forcefully pumping out air. This exercise is similar to the Abdominal Breath, but places greater concentration on the exhalation. Sit comfortably with your spine erect. Empty your lungs completely. Inhale through the nose, filling your lungs to approximately half their capacity, and at the same time pushing out your abdomen. Until you have more practice, keep your fingers lightly on your abdomen in order to be aware of abdominal movement. Very vigorously, exhale through the front of your nose as if you were blowing your nose (it's a good idea to have a tissue handy), simultaneously contracting the stomach muscles forcefully. Do ten Charging Breaths followed by one Complete Breath.

Start off slowly. Think of a train beginning slowly and gradually increasing in speed, chugging faster and faster. Increase the speed and number of breaths gradually with practice, adding ten more Charging Breaths at a time. Follow each set with a Complete Breath. After a few weeks, you should be able to do thirty Charging Breaths comfortably, between each Complete Breath. Be cautious not to exceed your capacity for you may get dizzy in the beginning.

You will experience immediate revitalization with this exercise, as you replenish your energy supply. This breathing can definitely result in a state of exhilaration. Former drug users have learned that they can "get high" naturally by prolonged practice of this exercise. They say they experience the same state of euphoria as with drugs, with a more lasting effect. I must emphasize that extensive practice of this technique should not be attempted without the aid of a competent instructor, as it may cause hyperventilation.

This practice empties and cleans the walls of the lungs of residue. It is especially recommended for smokers to help clean the lungs of nicotine. Nonsmokers will also find it beneficial in expelling the various pollutants to which we are constantly subjected, especially in urban areas. The Bellows Breath increases the supply of oxygen in the blood, producing the radiance of good health.

Glottis or Throat Breath

I recommend this technique as invaluable to every Yoga practitioner and to the serious athlete because it helps every activity to be more forceful and dynamic. It is also easier to use than the Abdominal or Complete Breath when twisting, turning and inverting in Yoga and other exercises, as well as in accelerated sports movement.

The glottis is a cleft between the vocal cords at the upper opening of the larynx. Picture it located in the middle of the throat in a line with the clavicle. You can discover its exact location when you imitate a slight snore or in clearing your throat.

Sit in a comfortable position with the spine straight. Expel all breath through the mouth. Relax the abdomen and breathe in through the nose by partially closing the glottis but keeping the nostrils relaxed and open. A sobbing sound should be produced by the breathing because of the partial closure of the glottis. Breathe out with your concentration on the glottis. Never hold the breath. Concentrate on rhythmic in and out movement. The abdomen and rib cage should not be involved in this routine; only the chest is activated. This breathing becomes a powerful chest exercise.

You will have to consciously concentrate on your Glottis Breathing as you combine this breath with your exercises and sports. It will become an uninhibited movement with time. The same holds true for the other breathing techniques. Ultimately, you will breathe as nature intended you to.

Exercises

Here is a basic program for beginners and intermediates. Whatever your level, work to your own capacity. You are not competing with anyone else. Follow the instructions to the best of your ability, don't set standards for yourself and don't be impatient. Remember that consistency of practice instead of achievement level should be your foremost concern, especially in the beginning. If you have never exercised, or are in poor shape or physical condition at present, start off with as few as five positions. Choose one warm-up exercise, one standing pose such as the Triangle, one sitting pose, perhaps the Alternate Leg Stretch. Lying on your back, practice the Shoulderstand against the wall and follow up with the Fish posture. Practice one back bend, either the Cobra, the Half Bow or the Half Locust. Finish with Complete Relaxation. Gradually add other poses to your program as you become stronger.

Beginners, I suggest you have a soft belt or a strap at your side as you start. It is used to extend your arm reach as you hold onto your knees, calves or feet, and is an invaluable tool to help you prevent undue straining or pulling of muscles. You can use any nonelasticized belt or strap that you have around the house. Have a small pillow handy to elevate your back if sitting straight on the floor is uncomfortable for you in the beginning. A folded, not too soft blanket, is helpful for relief and prevention of neck problems as you practice the Shoulderstand.

I urge all students to follow the sequence of exercises as pictured. Start by warming up your body, proceed into standing, sitting down, lying on back, and back-bending positions. It has been my experience during my many years of teaching that this particular routine of concave and convex movements leads to amazing results in flexibility and strength in the shortest period of time. Please coordinate your breathing with each pose. While exercising, you will breathe with concentration on the glottis or back of throat. Breathe in through the nose and out through the nose or the mouth, whichever is most comfortable for you. Don't concern yourself with expanding or contracting the abdomen. These movements will evolve naturally as you practice the other breathing techniques. It is physiologically correct to breathe in as you enter into the posture and breathe out as you relax into the stretch. But please don't be rigid and don't worry if you reverse the process. Right now, concentrate only on conscious breathing and you can do no wrong.

Before you start your practice, always sit or lie down with eyes closed for a few minutes. Mentally advise yourself that this is not just another exercise program to get out of the way. You are striving to function in healthy harmony, not just in body, but emotions, mind and spirit as well. Promise yourself to focus all your awareness and attention on your movements. Be aware that your thoughts may want to stray in other directions, but that you will bring them back gently to your present direction toward self-love and self-improvement. Be aware that you are working for yourself only, in what may be the most important undertaking of your life.

Knee to Chest Bend

This pose helps to stretch the lower back muscles and spine and prepares you for back-arching poses. It also strengthens the upper back and neck.

Beginner: Lie on the floor with feet on the floor and knees bent. Lift one leg and clasp hands below the knee. If you cannot grasp your knee comfortably, use your strap to extend your arm reach. Inhale, as you lift the head and press knee tightly to your chest. Exhale, hold ten seconds, relax. Do this twice and repeat on the other side.

Intermediate: Both legs are on the floor, straight. Bend one knee, clasp hands around knee. Roll up the head, touching the forehead to knee if possible, and squeeze the knee to chest. (Always follow beginner directions as to breathing, length of hold and number of repetitions for all poses.)

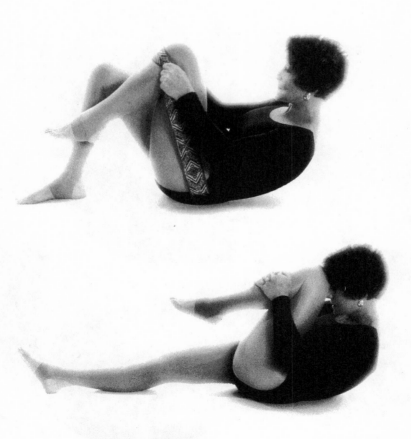

Leg to Chest Pose

Promotes flexibility in the back muscles of the entire leg as well as hips. It also strengthens the knees and upper back.

Beginner: Bend one leg at the knee, placing the foot firmly on the floor. Wrap the strap around the back of the other knee, calf, ankle or foot—wherever you can reach—but keep the knee straight. Inhale, lift the head as high as possible and pull the leg toward you. Exhale, hold ten seconds, relax. Do this twice and repeat on the other side.

Intermediate: Both legs are on the floor, straight. Raise one leg and firmly clasp the ankle, toes or foot. Raise the head and move the leg toward the forehead.

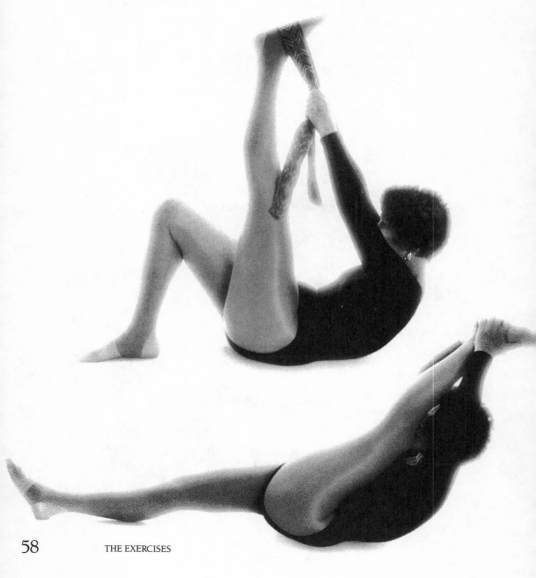

Bridge Pose

Loosens shoulder blades and strengthens the lower back and abdominal muscles.

Beginner: Lie down, arms at your sides, palms down. Bend the knees and place the feet close to your body. Feet are parallel and about twelve inches apart. Placing your weight on your buttocks, shoulders and head, inhale, raise your back one vertebra at a time, starting with the tailbone. Exhale. Keeping the weight on the shoulders, soften the back of the neck and gently press it into the floor. Expand the rib cage. Tighten the buttocks and raise the pelvis. Breathe normally, hold ten to thirty seconds. Inhaling, lower the back one vertebra at a time. Exhale. Press the small of the back into the floor for a count of eight before releasing the hips. Repeat.

Intermediate: Start in the beginner pose. When your back and buttocks are lifted, bend arms at elbows and place palms firmly into the small of the back. Slowly straighten the legs, one at a time. If you find this too difficult right now, keep your knees bent.

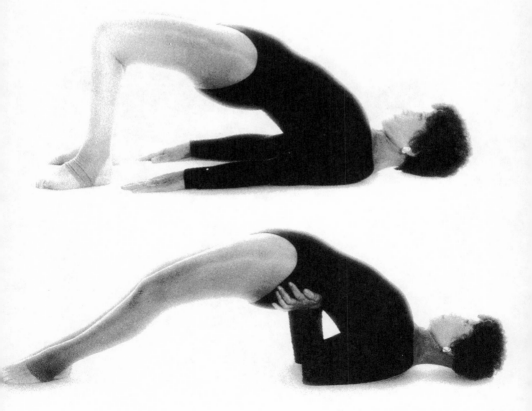

Spinal Stretch

Releases tension in, and stretches, the lower back. Also loosens hamstring muscles.

Beginner and Intermediate: If you like, you can hold on to an exercise bar or ledge as you do this exercise. Stand with feet slightly apart, placed underneath the hips. Bend forward and stretch the spine and arms to their capacity, keeping arms perpendicular to the floor. Make the lower back concave, and stretch into the coccyx and back of thighs. Breathe deeply and hold the pose for at least one minute.

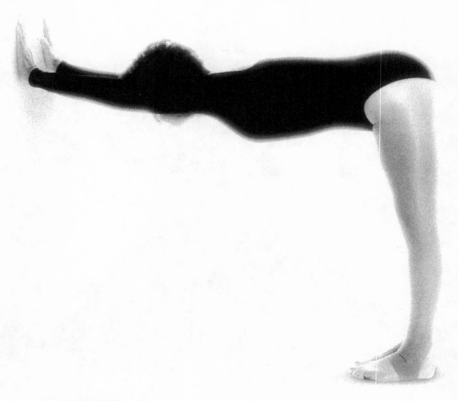

Forward Bend

Loosens and relaxes the lower spine. Especially helpful for lower back problems and to prevent injury.

Beginner and Intermediate: Press the lower back firmly against the wall and walk your feet away from you. Very slowly roll forward, head and neck followed by the upper back. Arms are hanging loosely. When you can bend no further, hold onto your elbows and relax into the position. Relax your head and neck and breathe deeply. Hold one minute or longer. If you have lower back problems, hold this position twice a day for five minutes. Let the arms dangle and roll up very slowly.

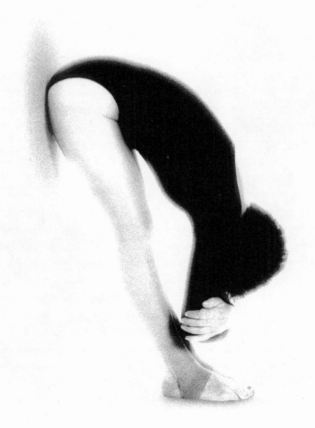

Chest Expansion

Loosens shoulders, neck and upper back. Widens thoracic area. Elongates spine and hamstring muscles and promotes superb spinal flexibility.

Beginner: Feet are about ten inches apart. Interlace fingers firmly behind your back. Lift arms as high as possible, keeping them straight. Inhale and bend forward slowly, leading with the head. Exhale. Relax the spine, shoulders and head but continue to straighten the arms. Hold ten to thirty seconds, breathing naturally. Roll up slowly. Do twice.

Intermediate: Feet are touching, hands interlace behind back. Try to raise arms to shoulder level, keeping them straight. Bend forward with straight back, leading with the head. Round the back when you need to, and move the torso toward the knees. The legs remain straight.

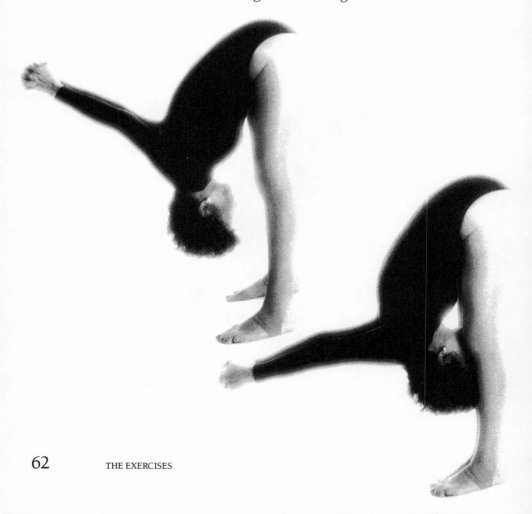

Triangle Pose

This pose increases balance. It tones and strengthens the legs, waist, abdomen, hips, chest, shoulders and arms. It promotes lateral flexibility of the upper torso.

Beginner: Place the feet about three feet apart and parallel to each other. Raise arms to the sides, shoulder level with the palms down. Turn the left foot in and the right foot to the side. Simultaneously move the left hip directly to the side, inhale and slide the right hand down the right leg as far as you can without turning the torso and pelvis. Stretch left hand toward the ceiling. Exhale. Inhale, rotate the torso toward the back and look at your upstretched hand, exhale. Do once, hold the position as long as possible. Move up slowly. Repeat on the other side.

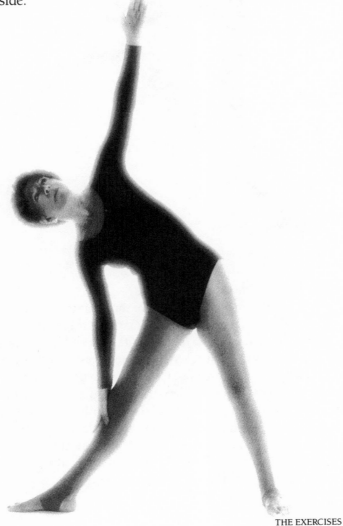

Intermediate: Legs are about five feet apart. Slide the hand down the leg as far as you can reach, holding on to the ankle or possibly placing the hand on the floor. Do not sacrifice straightness of torso or legs. With an inhale, move the out-stretched arm in line with your ear. Exhale.

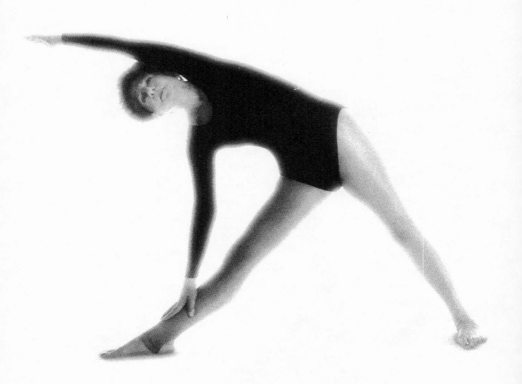

Reversed Triangle Pose

This is an excellent rotation for the lateral spine. It strengthens the spine and back muscles, and tones thigh and calf muscles and hamstrings. It invigorates the abdominal organs, strengthens the hip muscles and slenderizes the waistline.

Beginner: Legs are about three feet apart. Turn the left foot in and the right foot out. Place the left arm around the back of the waistline, turn your torso to the left. Inhale as you slide the right hand down the right thigh to the knee. Clasp firmly and exhale. With another inhale gently twist your torso toward the back. Exhale. Breathe in and out as you are holding the pose to prevent strain. Hold as long as you can and move out of the position very slowly.

Intermediate: Separate the legs to three and a half feet, raise arms to the sides at shoulder level. Turn the left foot in and the right foot to the side. Tighten and stretch the leg muscles, pressing the heel and outer sole onto the floor (do not lose the leg stance as you continue). Twist the torso to the right, placing the left hand outside the right foot or gripping the leg wherever possible. Keeping the right arm straight, gaze at the right hand, and stretch the arms and shoulders intensely.

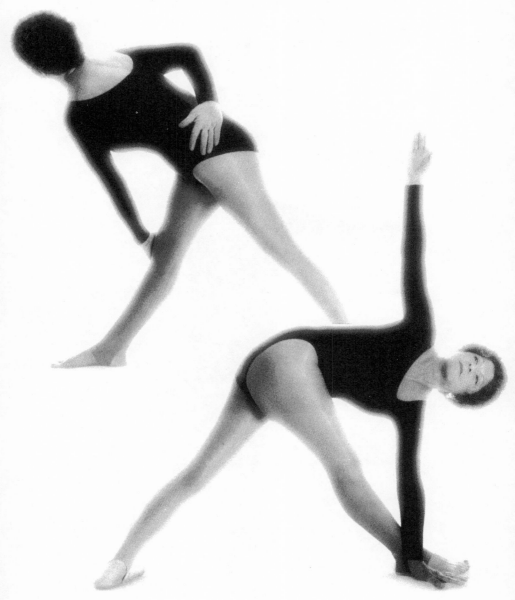

Stork Pose

This position will enhance your ability to balance. It tones the leg muscles, especially the inner thighs, and slenderizes the torso.

Beginner: Balance on one foot. Bending the other leg at the knee, hold onto the ankle and slide the foot up the inner leg toward the groin. Hold wherever you can. You may only reach the inner knee at this time, but don't be discouraged. Extend your other arm to the side and breathe evenly. If you are very unsteady, place your fingertips on a wall. Hold as long as possible, repeat on the other side.

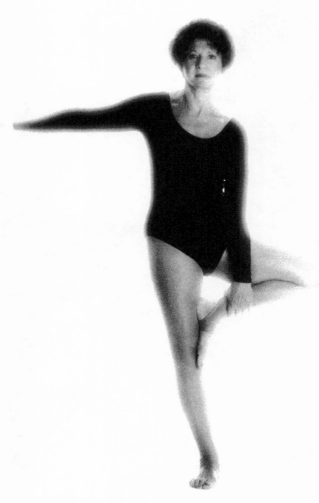

Intermediate: Press the foot into the thigh and with equal pressure, press the thigh against the foot, to stay firmly locked. Raise the arms slowly above the head, tighten every muscle in the body and hold at least two minutes. Concentrate on the breath — this will facilitate your balance.

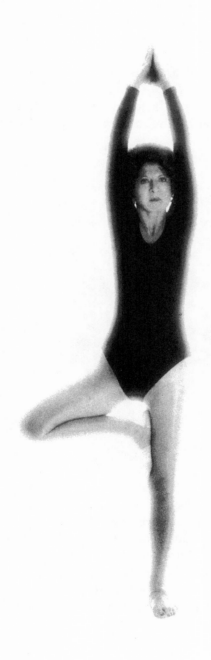

Sit down as gracefully as possible.

Cradle Rock

To loosen the knee joints.

Beginner and Intermediate: Beginners may want to elevate their backs, sitting not on, but at the edge of a pillow. Bend one leg at the knee, placing the foot against the inner thigh of the opposite leg. Clasp your hands around the other knee and the foot, interlacing the hands in the center if possible. Sit straight, inhale and press the knee to or toward the chest. Exhale and hold. Repeat twice more. Release knee from chest and, still holding it with your clasped hands, move the leg from side to side; make believe that you are rocking a baby. Repeat on the other side.

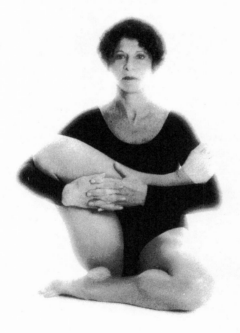

Alternate Leg Stretch

The Alternate Leg Stretch is one of the best positions for restoring flexibility, elasticity and youthfulness to any spine in any condition. The hold also benefits the legs, stretching muscles, ligaments and tendons. It relieves stiffness and tension, especially in the back of the legs. It firms the entire body, especially the legs, thighs, buttocks, hips and abdomen.

Beginner: Bend one knee and move the foot toward the inner thigh of the opposite leg. You may only reach the inner knee in the beginning. Place your strap around the other foot and sit straight. Inhale and very slowly bend forward, leading from the lower back. Exhale. Do not allow your back to round, even if you can only move a few inches at this time. Breathe normally, holding the position for twenty seconds. Do not strain; your back will loosen when it is ready. Repeat on same side and twice on the other side.

Intermediate: Sit with legs straight in front of you. With both hands, pick up one foot and guide the heel into the perineum wth the sole against the thigh. Keep both knees on the floor and the back straight. Lift your arms to the side and over the head, clasp thumbs and stretch to your capacity. Inhale, come forward with a straight back, and exhale. Firmly grasp your ankle or place the hands around the foot. Bending elbows outward and keeping shoulders back and down, slide your torso forward, bringing the rib cage toward the thigh. For added flexibility place your head on the floor. Breathe normally, and continue to stretch without strain. Hold one minute at the first stretch and two minutes the second time on each side.

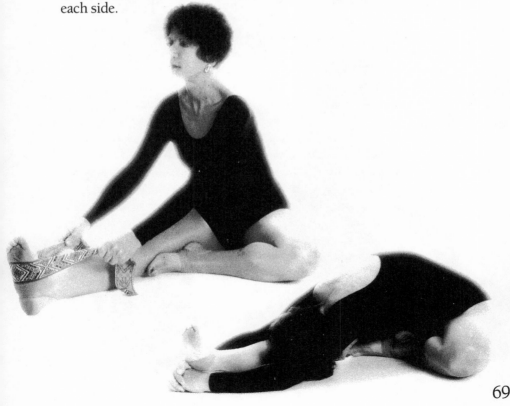

Complete Leg Stretch

Offers the same benefits as the Alternate Leg Stretch, but with greater emphasis on stretching the hamstring muscles, the stiffest muscles in the legs. Because the hamstring muscles are coordinated with the lower back muscles, you will be simultaneously loosening your lower back as you do this exercise. The Complete Leg Stretch is also a powerful aid for firming the legs, waist, abdomen and hips.

Beginner: Sit erect, bend the legs and slide your strap under your feet. Slowly straighten the legs along the floor. Holding the strap firmly, pull the elbows toward your back if possible, in order to maintain a straight spine. Breathe in as you bend forward. Exhale as you reach your utmost stretch. Don't round the spine, and keep the knees straight. Hold for at least one minute. Build up to holding the position for three minutes. Do once.

Intermediate: Sit erect, with legs extended straight in front of you and hands on thighs. Slowly raise both arms to the side, then above your head. Clasp your thumbs, stretch, and inhale. Exhaling, come forward slowly, stretching from the lower back and leading with the rib cage. Grip firmly whatever part of your legs you can reach, calves, ankles, or feet. Bending the elbows, pull your torso forward. Avoid rounding the upper back. Breathe normally and hold for three to five minutes.

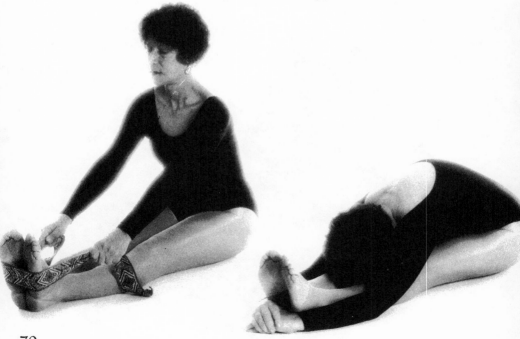

Inner Thigh Stretch or Butterfly

Loosens knees and ankles. Tones and tightens inner thighs and helps to straighten spine.

Beginner (Butterfly): Sit erect, place the soles of the feet together and push the feet toward the groin as far as they will go. Holding your feet with your hands, flap the knees up and down, slowly at first and increasing the speed in coordination with your breathing. Notice how you are loosening the knee joints and the inner thigh muscles.

Intermediate (Inner Thigh Stretch): Sit erect. Place the soles of your feet together and pull the feet toward the groin. Do not allow the spine to round. Inhale deeply. Exhaling slowly, bring your knees toward the floor as you continue to hold your feet with your hands. Don't be afraid to push down as far as possible. You can't hurt the knees in this position. Breathe normally and hold the extreme position for at least thirty seconds. Perform three times.

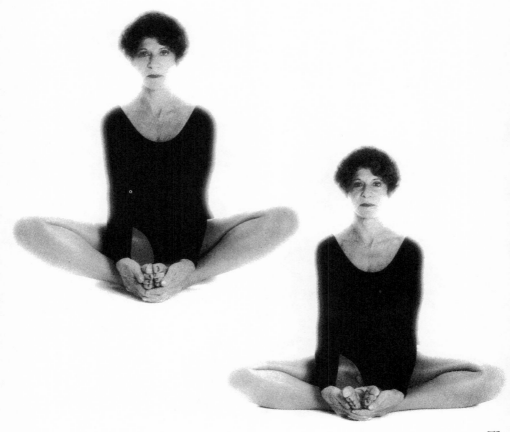

Sitting Twist

By locking the lower part of your body, you're free to twist the upper body to its utmost, enabling you to get rid of back pains, strains, kinks and general discomfort. Spinal flexibility is greatly improved. Twisting in this way helps take inches from the waist. You will experience immediate invigoration.

Beginner: With your right leg straight in front of you, bend your left knee and place the left foot on the floor next to the outer thigh of the right leg. Place your left hand firmly on the floor behind you, in line with your lower back. Take your right hand to the back of the left knee and push the knee backward as far as possible. Sitting ramrod straight, inhale and twist over your left shoulder. Exhale and hold the position for at least ten seconds. Twist twice on same side and repeat on the other side.

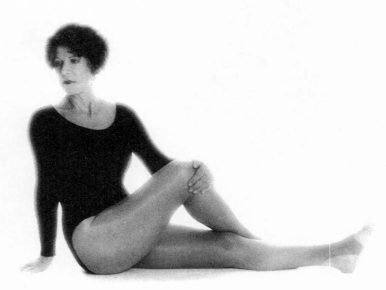

Intermediate: First position – Bend your left leg to the groin as in the Alternate Leg Stretch. Bend the right leg, clasp the hands around the knee and place the foot to stand in back of the bent knee. Bend your left arm, reaching across your torso, and with the elbow push the knee away from you. The right hand is placed on the floor behind you, in line with the lower back. Inhale as you twist over your right shoulder, exhale and hold for at least thirty seconds. Twist twice on same side and repeat.

Second Position – When you are flexible enough to attempt this pose, slide the left arm through the leg. Circle the right arm around the back, and with an inhale try to clasp the hands or preferably the wrist. Exhale as you twist. Hold for at least one minute.

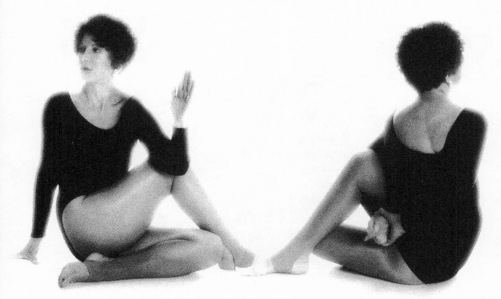

Lie down carefully.

Knees to Chest Pose

This simple movement will release all tension from the lower back muscles and spine and prepare you for the inversions of the Shoulderstand and Plough and the ensuing back-bending positions.

Beginner and Intermediate: On your back, bring the knees to the chest, clasp your hands around the knees or just hold on to the knees. Inhale, and firmly squeeze the knees into the chest. Exhale, and hold tightly for at least ten seconds. Release and repeat twice more. You can also rock gently back and forth or from side to side.

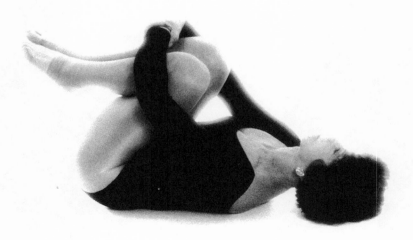

Shoulderstand

We are now ready for the Shoulderstand. This position is considered to be of maximum therapeutic value for almost every person. Those suffering from severe hypertension, cardiovascular disorders or extreme obesity should either proceed with great caution, or skip it altogether. I am listing only a few of the multitude of benefits that this position has to offer: The blood is able to flow freely throughout the entire body, stimulating organs and glands, especially the thyroid and parathyroid. The increased blood supply to the brain combats fatigue, tones up the nervous system and prevents senility. The spine becomes strong and pain free. The visceral organs are relieved from the constant pull of gravity, and digestive disorders can be corrected.

Beginner: This exercise requires a wall to help you get into position. Use your blanket or even two blankets if your neck and shoulders are weak. Place the blanket next to the wall. Manipulate yourself to place the shoulders on the rolled edge of the blanket with your head resting loosely on the floor. The lower back is touching the wall and your legs are straight up against the wall. Bend the knees and push the soles of the feet firmly into the wall. Lift your lower back away from the wall and support it immediately with the palms of the hands

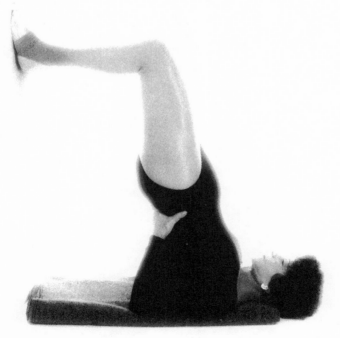

meeting in the middle, keeping your feet on the wall. The elbows are resting on the floor. Try to keep them close together. Hold the position as long as possible, breathing slowly and rhythmically. Lower yourself carefully. Remain for a few seconds with the spine against the wall and the legs straight up the wall. Bend the knees toward your head, roll to one side and sit up slowly. When your back becomes stronger, you can attempt to straighten the legs against the wall while you are supporting your spine. Eventually you may try to move your legs away from the wall, one leg at a time.

Intermediate: This exercise does not use a wall to help you get into position. Lie on the floor with legs straight together, arms close to the body, palms of the hands down. Pressing arms and hands against the floor, raise your legs while contracting the abdomen. When your legs are perpendicular to the floor, inhale quickly, raising the hips and buttocks and

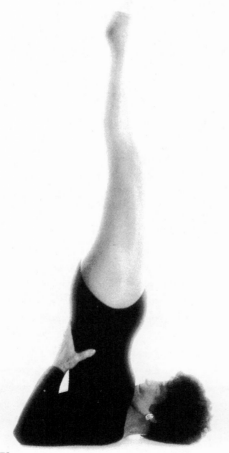

placing your hands on the lower spine for support. Gradually move your hands up your spine and move your elbows closer together, eventually reaching the extreme position with legs and body as straight as a candle. Thighs, inner knees, ankles and soles should be touching, with legs and spine stretching toward the ceiling. Press your chin into the jugular notch for added stimulation of the thyroid gland. Try to hold the position for three minutes, breathing normally. As your back becomes stronger, try moving your hands toward the floor and interlocking them as pictured in the Plough position.

It is important that you roll out of the Shoulderstand carefully to avoid hurting your spine. Bend your knees to rest on the top of the forehead. Either supporting your back or placing the palms flat on the floor, arch your neck and upper back and proceed to lower yourself very slowly. Feel each vertebra touching the floor as you roll down. This is a wonderful massage and stimulation for your entire spinal column.

Plough Pose

This exercise stretches the spine for maximum flexibility and rejuvenation. It is a very important pose to strengthen all dorsal muscles. The Plough firms the hips, thighs and abdomen, while helping to subtract inches from these areas. It can provide almost immediate relief from tension and headaches. Arthritis and backache sufferers have reported the greatest relief from practicing this posture.

Beginner: Attempt the Plough only when you are able to move the legs away from the wall as you remain in the Shoulderstand. Get into the Shoulderstand position with your legs away from the wall. Supporting your back firmly, bend the knees and rest them on your forehead. Breathe rhythmically and effortlessly. Hold the position as long as you are able to without strain or pain. Do not be in a hurry to straighten the legs; this will come about as soon as your spine allows it.

Intermediate: You may go into the Plough from the Shoulderstand by keeping the spine straight and lowering the legs toward the floor behind the head. Or you may enter into it the same way as in the Shoulderstand, keeping the legs straight, bending at the waist and placing the feet on the floor in back of you. Continue to straighten the spine, and push the bones of the buttocks up toward the ceiling. If your back is strong, walk the legs as close to your head as possible while elongating the spine. You may interlock your hands on the floor to take the pressure off your neck. Concentrate on the breath as you hold the pose for at least three minutes. Roll out carefully as from the Shoulderstand. It is a good idea for everybody to once more go into the Knees to Chest pose to release all residue of tension.

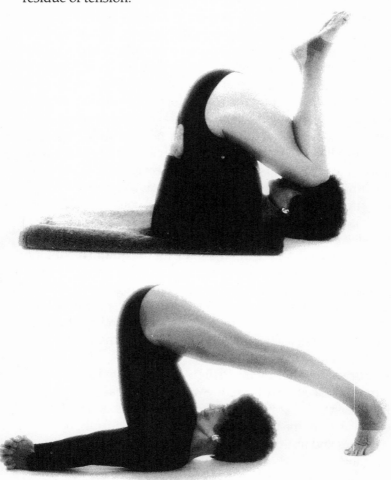

Fish Pose

(I always wondered why the position was thus named, and I recently learned that one can float on the surface of water in this pose. I haven't tried it as yet.) This posture is of great cosmetic value to both men and women, preventing crepe neck and double chins by firming the muscles. (This I can vouch for!) It is a counterbalance to the Shoulderstand and the Plough, arching the spine in the opposite direction. It also stimulates the thyroid gland and acts as an overall tonic to the nervous system.

Beginner: Lie on your back, with legs straight out in front of you and arms at your sides. Place the hands under the buttocks with palms up and raise your upper back and head from the floor. Square your shoulders and arch your upper back, letting the head hang limply. Placing all the weight on your hands, slowly lower the back of the head to the floor, while stretching the neck and expanding the chest. Breathe deeply into the throat area and feel the chest opening up and the back muscles relaxing. Hold thirty seconds to one minute and slowly roll out.

Intermediate: Don't attempt this position until your legs have become flexible and your spine is strong. Lie on your back, bend your knees, cross your legs and fold your feet under your buttocks. Hold on to your feet or, if possible, your ankles. Arch the upper part of your body, letting your weight rest on your head, elbows and feet. Arch your thighs and hips, and try to have the knees touch the floor. Breathe deeply, while holding the position for a minute or so.

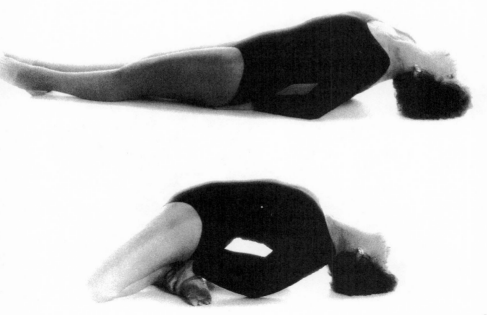

Wheel Pose

This is another convex pose to be alternated with or performed in addition to the Fish Pose. It is a very powerful exercise, especially in the intermediate version, for strengthening the thighs, buttocks, upper back, shoulder and arm muscles. The high arch in the extreme version promotes utmost flexibility for the lower back. It is perhaps the most energizing of all the postures.

Beginner: Sit up, bend your knees and place your hands, palms down, directly in back of you. The hands are about twelve inches away from your body, fingers pointing to the back, and the elbows are locked. Separate your feet to the same distance as the hands. Press the soles of the feet firmly into the floor, and with an inhale raise the lower torso off the floor. Exhale. Tighten your thighs, buttocks and abdominals. Take another breath, expand the chest and push it toward the ceiling. Exhale and relax the head. Hold as long as you can, breathing evenly. Lower yourself slowly.

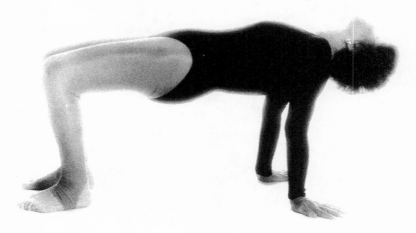

Intermediate: Lie on your back and walk the feet close to the buttocks. Legs are about ten inches apart. Place the palms on the floor directly under the shoulders, fingers pointing toward the feet. Take a deep breath, and pushing hard on the feet and hands, raise the hips and the chest, arching toward the ceiling. Exhale, and continue with rhythmic breathing. Hold as long as you can and come down carefully. This may be a very strenuous position at first try, but if you continue, the back will loosen. After the fifth push-up, this pose actually becomes fun to do.

You will now shift your position from lying on your back. Generally speaking, whenever you get up from lying on your back, please proceed carefully and sensibly. This is important even for those who are free from back problems. Roll to one side and bend your knees to your chest. Placing the hands in front of the shoulders, slowly come to all fours. Stretch for a moment before you stand, sit or roll over. This is also a good way to get out of bed in the morning.

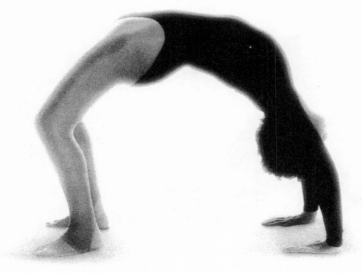

Cobra Pose

The Cobra stretches all the vertebrae, especially those of the upper back and neck, promoting flexibility and generally toning the spine and sympathetic nervous system. Accumulated tension in the upper back and neck is relieved. Posture is improved. All the inner organs are massaged, stimulating the action of these organs for general good health. Muscles in the abdomen, bust and chest are firmed. The Cobra provides fresh vitality, yet it induces sleep in case of insomnia.

Beginner: Lie on your abdomen, wth arms stretched over your head and legs straight, feet and hands slightly apart, palms facing the floor. Tighten the legs, buttocks and abdomen, inhale, and walk your hands toward you as you lift and arch your head, shoulders and upper torso. Be cautious if you have lower back problems. Allow your back to let you know when to stop. In the completed pose the arms are straight with elbows locked and the shoulders relaxed. Stretch the neck and let the head roll back slightly. Breathe normally and hold the pose for at least thirty seconds. Walk the hands down the same way, one hand at a time, with arms remaining straight as you lower your torso and head to the floor. Rest for a few seconds and repeat one more time. All poses performed lying on your stomach are especially strenuous. It is advisable that you rest after each pose. Make a pillow with your hands and turn your head to the side. Close your eyes and breathe evenly.

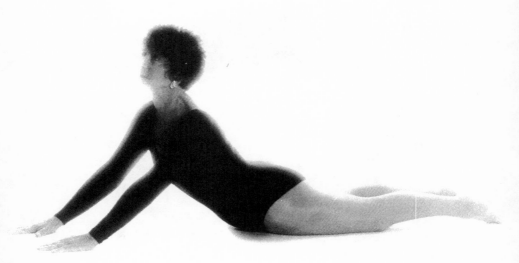

Intermediate: Place your hands directly under your chest, arms in line with the shoulders, forehead to the ground. The lower body is tightly locked. Inhale, and in a succession of flowing movements, lift up your chin, roll back your head, stretch the upper torso forward, and raise your shoulders. Keeping the pelvis on the floor and the head back, continue pushing yourself up slowly, until the arms are straight. Exhale whenever you have to. Shoulders are relaxed, neck stretched and head rolled back as far as possible. The feet, knees and thighs should be touching in the completed pose. Come out of the position by bending your elbows and slowly lowering your body, keeping your head back as long as possible. Your chin is the last part of the body to reach the floor. Relax and repeat.

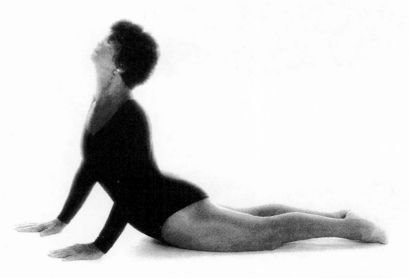

Locust Pose

In this position, the muscles of the lower body and the arms are subjected to strong tension, resulting in firming of the upper arms, abdomen, hips, buttocks and thighs. The sex organs and glands are greatly stimulated in this pose. The Locust strengthens the lower back area, with emphasis on the sacroiliac. All visceral organs and glands are stimulated as well, relieving digestive disorders.

Beginner (Half Locust): Lie on your stomach, with arms at your sides, chin on the floor and feet together. Make fists and bring your entire arms under you with fists under your thighs, so that the body is supported by the arms. Your fists can be up or down, whichever way provides the best balance. Inhale. With chin pressing into the floor, raise one leg straight up and exhale. The knee is locked. Inhale again and try to lift the leg higher, keeping the body aligned. Exhale, stretch for another five seconds and lower the leg slowly. Repeat and do twice on the other side.

Intermediate (Full Locust): Prepare for the position as in the beginner version. With fists pressed firmly against the floor, inhale and lift both legs quickly, then exhale. Inhale and make an effort to raise the legs higher. Exhale, hold for about ten seconds and lower legs very slowly.

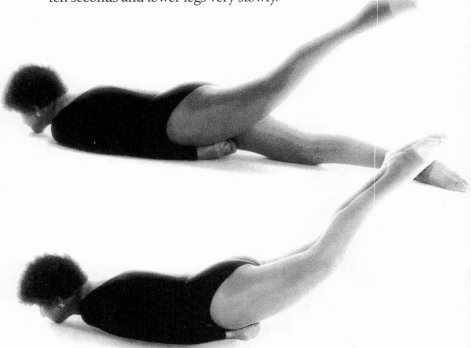

Bow Pose

The Bow strengthens and develops the entire spine, resulting in complete elasticity. It firms the whole body, with emphasis on upper arms, bust, hips, buttocks and thighs. It improves posture and helps to relieve menstrual disorders and lower-back pain. It can also greatly relieve physical and mental tension.

Beginner (Half Bow): While the bow is designed to make your back strong, you must proceed with caution in the beginning. Whenever your body tells you to stop, you must listen to it. Lie on your abdomen, arms at your sides and legs straight. Bend one arm at the elbow and place the hand under your chest. Bend the opposite leg and with the other hand take hold of the ankle. If you cannot reach the ankle, do not hold on to the toes, but use your strap instead. With an inhale, pressing the lower arm firmly into the floor, raise the upper body and try to lift the thigh off the floor. Exhale. If the thigh will not move as yet, don't be impatient. The groin muscles, which are responsible, will loosen up in no time at all. Hold five seconds, repeat on same side and twice on the other side.

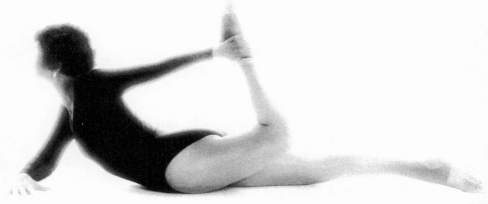

Intermediate (Full Bow): Lie on abdomen, thighs apart and chin on the floor. Bring your heels up toward your back. Reach back and firmly grasp your ankles. (If you cannot reach your ankles, you are not ready for this pose. Practice the Half Bow instead.) Inhale and raise your head, shoulders and chest off the floor, then exhale. Inhale again and lift your thighs as high as possible, exhale and arch into a perfect bow with feet together. Eventually your thighs will touch the floor and your feet will be together. Hold as long as possible and repeat. Don't forget to rest in between these exercises.

To move out of the lying-down positions, place your hands under the shoulders. Very slowly straighten your arms and push on to your knees. Think of yourself as a cat stretching after a nap. Come to sit on your heels.

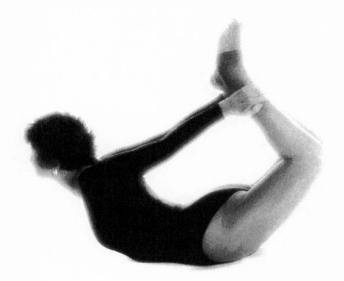

Child Pose

This is an excellent rest position to perform after an exercise session or whenever you feel tired or tense. It stretches all the muscles in the back and releases pain, strain and tension in the feet.

Beginner and Intermediate: While sitting on your heels, lengthen the abdomen, bend forward and rest the abdomen on the thighs. The head touches either the floor or the knees and the arms rest loosely at the sides. Focus on deep rhythmic breathing and relax for at least twenty seconds.

Slowly sit up, shift to sit to one side of the knees, straighten your legs, and very carefully lie down. You are now ready for Complete Relaxation. You may want to tape this section and let your own voice guide you as you relax. Speak softly and slowly, and when the tape shuts off continue to lie quietly for a little while longer.

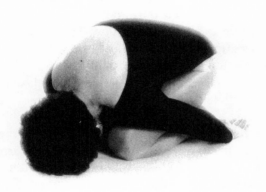

Complete Relaxation

Lie on your back on a flat surface with arms at your sides, slightly separated from the body, palms turned up. The legs are parted as well, feet turned outward. The shoulders are relaxed and so is the neck. Rotate your head slowly from side to side until you find a comfortable position for it. Close your eyes and say to yourself: "I am now ready to relax completely. My body is becoming limp and light, and all tension and strain is leaving me. My joints are loose and all muscles are relaxed. I am not doing anything right now, I have given up all effort and I am turning deep within myself, into the innermost recesses of my being, where lies rest, peace and tranquility. My body is the temple of the spirit. It is healthy and strong, firm and flexible, pure as a crystal, soft and supple and graceful as a flower. My mind is relaxed, calm, clear and lucid. I am letting go of all worries, speculations, expectations, and all thoughts of the past and the future. I am in the present only, and my thoughts have been suspended. I breathe in deeply, and as I exhale I let my body sink into the floor in total relaxation. Again I inhale deeply, and as I exhale I empty my mind of all thought and all conscious effort. Once more I inhale deeply and with the exhalation I become aware of both my body and mind entering into a blissful state of complete relaxation.

I now focus on my right foot. I relax the toes, one by one, until they are soft and limp. I relax the sole of the foot, the arch and the instep. I now relax the ankle and let the relaxation move up into the calf and shin, the kneecap and the back of the knee, through the thigh into the groin. Now I forget about my right leg and concentrate only on the left foot. I relax the toes, the sole, arch and instep and follow the sensation of relaxation as it moves upward. It is flowing through the ankle, the shin and calf, the kneecap and back of the knee, the thigh and the groin. Both legs are now completely, deeply relaxed. They are heavy and still. I let them go and become aware of my right hand only. I relax all the fingers, one by one, all the joints and bones and knuckles. I relax the palm and the back of the hand. I relax the wrist, the lower arm, the elbow, the upper arm and the shoulder. I now devote all my attention to my left hand. I relax all the fingers, one by one, all joints and knuckles, the inside and back of the hand. I allow the relaxation to move up into the wrist, lower arm, elbow, upper arm and shoulder. I am now aware of both arms, lying heavy and limp, almost as if detached from the rest of the body. The shoulders are completely relaxed, free from all strain and tension. I forget about the arms and shoulders and shift my attention to the bottom of my spine. I tell my whole lower back to relax. I consciously relax the coccyx and the sacrum and let the relaxation flood the lumbar area of my spine. I allow the relaxation to travel up the spine through the thoracic and the cervical back, all the way up into the atlas, the last vertebra of the spine. I tell all the vertebrae and all the discs between the vertebrae to relax and I consciously relax every muscle of the back. I observe the sense of relaxation flowing through the shoulders into the front of the torso. It is now entering the clavicle and moving downward. I follow the movement through the sternum, the chest, the rib cage, the waist, the area of the navel. The relaxation is moving through the belly into the abdominal area, reaching also the hips, the pelvis and the pubis.

The whole torso is now completely, deeply relaxed. It is heavy, still and sinking. I let go of the torso; it is no longer part of me. I am now aware only of the neck and the head. I relax all the muscles, tissues and bones of the neck. I relax all sides

of the neck and the inside of the neck and the inside of the
neck, the throat, larynx and glottis. The head is heavy and resting against the floor. I relax the back of the head and feel the
relaxation flowing through the scalp, into the forehead and the
temples. It is now travelling downward, relaxing the brows
and eyes. The eyeballs are sinking heavily into their sockets;
the lids are resting softly against the eyes. I feel the cheeks
relax, the ears, the nose, the lips, the chin and the jaw. The
inside of the mouth is relaxed as well, the teeth and the gums
are relaxed and the tongue is hanging loosely in the lower jaw.
The neck is soft, the head relaxed and the face is calm, tranquil
and serene. I now visualize my inner organs—the stomach,
intestines, liver, kidneys, bladder, spleen, diaphragm, heart
and lungs—being utterly relaxed. They are strong and healthy
and functioning in perfect harmony. The nerves are quiet and
calm. The heart is beating regularly and perfectly. The lungs
are breathing deeply, fully and rhythmically. The blood is cir-
culating freely and healthily throughout all the veins, arteries
and capillaries.

I now relax my whole body, the legs, arms, torso, neck
and head and the inner organs. The whole body is completely,
deeply relaxed. There is no tension, strain, pain, rigidity or discomfort in any part of my body. My mind is relaxed as well,
free from all pressure and all thought. I now allow my body
and mind to merge into one, to sink away, melt and dissolve
into a vast, blissful ocean of light. I let myself go deeper and
deeper into this all-encompassing, beautiful ocean of light. I
feel at one with the universe, one with the infinite spirit."

The following photos demonstrate what can be achieved through diligent practice by someone in her sixties who never exercised until age forty, and who had an inflexible, pain-ridden body to boot.

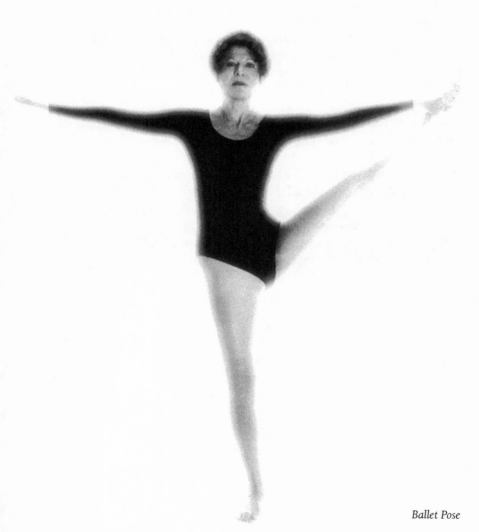

Ballet Pose

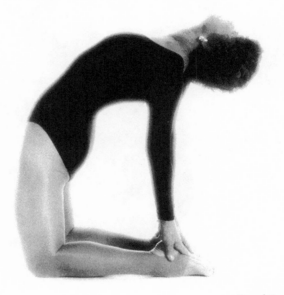

Camel Pose

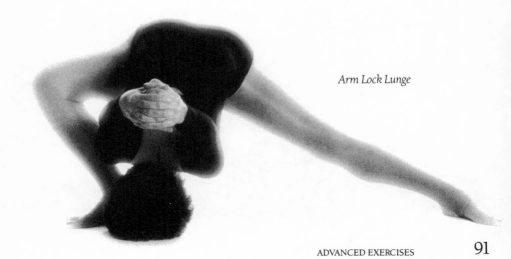

Arm Lock Lunge

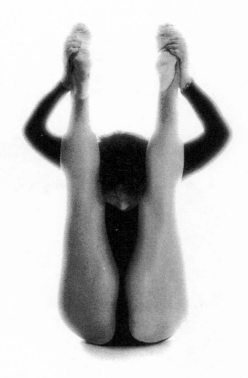

Hip Stand

Advanced Plough, variation

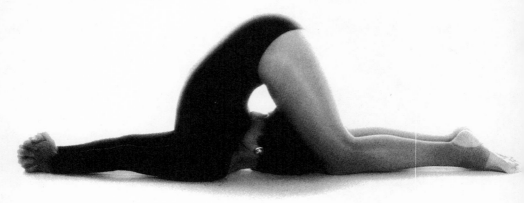

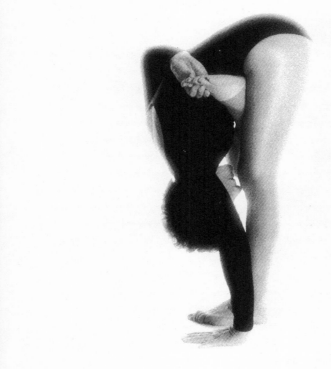

Tree, head to knee variation

Peacock Pose

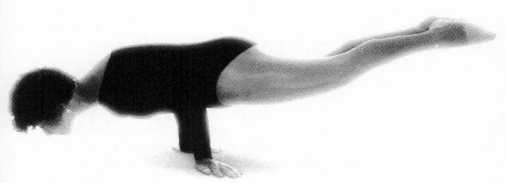

ADVANCED EXERCISES

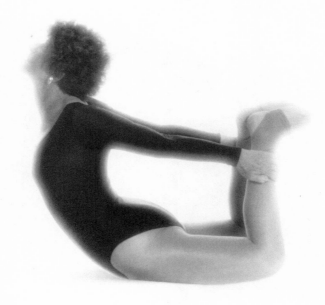

Advanced Bow Pose

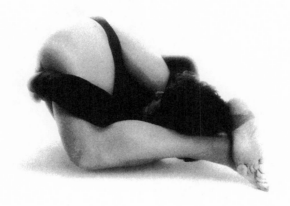

Noose Position

Extreme Chest Expansion

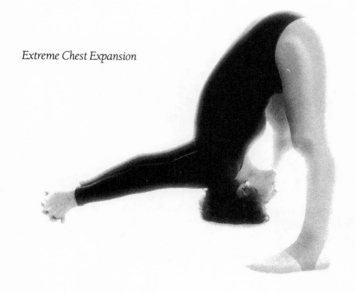

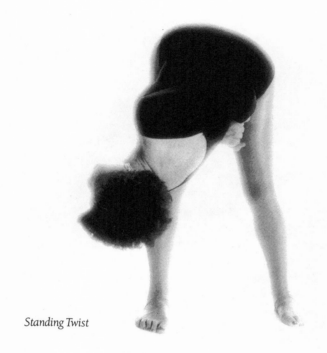

Standing Twist

Knee to Shoulder Plough

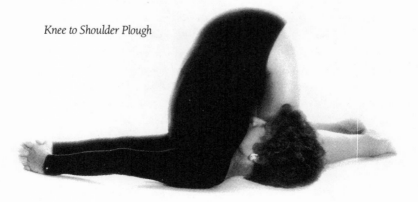

ADVANCED EXERCISES

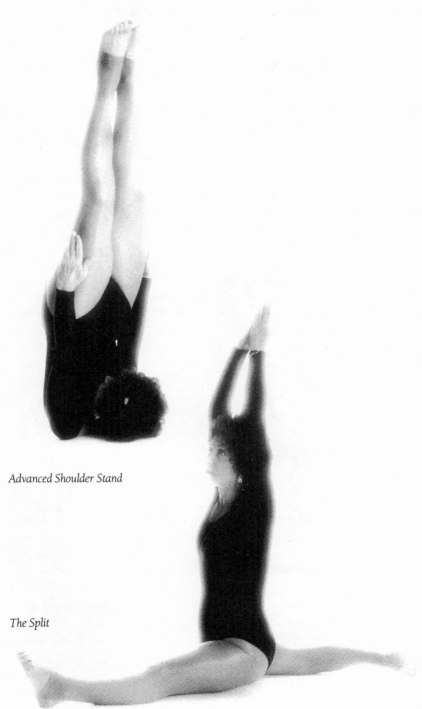

Advanced Shoulder Stand

The Split

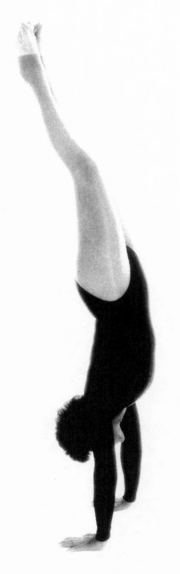

Handstand

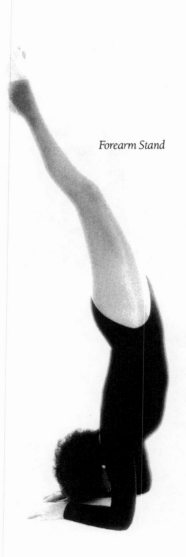

Forearm Stand

ADVANCED EXERCISES

CHAPTER FIVE

Common Sense Nutrition

A History of Nutrition in the United States

With the end of World War II, Americans experienced a radical change in eating habits. Many war casualties, we learned, were caused by nutritional deficiencies. Our soldiers suffered from anemia, bleeding gums, ulcers and a slew of intestinal and digestive diseases, attributed to their diet of Spam, powdered eggs, soda crackers and whiskey, and to lack of vitamins. The civilian population also seemed inadequately nourished. As one result, the vitamin industry was born and grew into a most lucrative enterprise. The study of dietetics was also begun. Licensed dieticians took charge of national nutrition. All efforts emphasized proper food balance and minimum daily requirements. The intake of vitamins, minerals, protein, amino acids, enzymes, carbohydrates and fatty acids was declared essential to good health and officially approved by the FDA. The dietician, who was appointed the authority in charge of menus for hospitals, school cafeterias, and public functions, strictly followed FDA guidelines.

A nutritious, balanced hospital or school lunch consisted of canned fruit juice, macaroni and cheese, canned string-beans, white bread and butter, Jell-o, and milk or coffee. Canned fruit cocktail, meat loaf with gravy, rice or potatoes, preserved peas, biscuits with butter, ice cream or pie for dessert — accompanied by lots of ice water and coffee — was the standard fare for banquets as well as the typical dinner for well-fed citizens. The ultimate in American cuisine was the steak dinner. For those who could afford it, and many could at the time, a true gourmet meal consisted of shrimp cocktail, steak smothered in onions, baked potato with butter and sour cream, a salad of iceberg lettuce with roquefort dressing, and cherries jubilee or baked Alaska for dessert. A southern meal featuring chicken and gravy, spoonbread, fritters and pecan pie would be equivalent in caloric content.

Afternoon and dinner cocktails were common, and the three-martini lunch became a part of the establishment. Food was the favorite pastime of the fabulous fifties. Everyone ate, drank and enjoyed, secure in the knowledge that America was the best-fed nation in the world and therefore the healthiest.

Young mothers relied on Dr. Spock to guide their infants' nutrition, and babies apparently thrived on milk formulas and Gerber's baby food. Mothers made sure that their older children had their orange juice, four glasses of milk and their one-a-day vitamin every day. The vitamin industry flourished. So did the breakfast cereal makers, inventing more inviting sugar-coated, frosted, multi-colored, attractively packaged toasties, crispies and wheaties to captivate the kiddies. Increased television advertising promoted snacks to accompany television viewing. Commercial breaks provided the cues to bring out potato chips, pretzels, crunchies, Coke and beer. TV dinners were presented as nutritious, balanced and swell.

Of all seven essential nutrients, protein was heralded as the most valuable. Protein, synonymous with meat, was considered to be the only food that contained all the necessary amino acids. Red meat was said to be the most healthful, so we made sure we had enough beef; steaks for the rich, hamburgers for the not-so-rich. Our diet did not include much grain except for white rice, because it was assumed that our need for carbohydrates was met by bread and breakfast cereals. Sugar was applauded as the finest source of carbohydrates for quick energy. A minimum of fresh fruits and vegetables were eaten. It was easier and cheaper to cope with canned or frozen produce, touted as being just as high in vitamin and mineral content and posing no spoilage problem. Because pesticides eradicated disease-carrying pests and strongly reduced crop losses, farmers were able to mass produce, but could not sell all their products. Wheat and other grains were given away to hungry nations or else burned. Many fruits and vegetables rotted.

In 1962, Rachel Carson, in her book *The Silent Spring,* claimed that we were being poisoned en masse and produced a national outrage against pesticides and pollutants. Yet that very panic proved to be favorable for the processed food industries which somehow managed to convince us that packaged, preserved, frozen, and canned foods ran less risk of contamination than natural produce. As the farmer went on growing food that was discarded, the fast food manufacturers thrived.

A drastic change in our attitudes toward food came about in the late sixties, together with all the other revolutions of the young and socially conscious. Their protests forced us to think about political issues, living standards and the dangers of environmental and food poisoning. Communes and co-ops were organized to produce pure, unadulterated foods. The public was made aware that we were being harmed by the chemical fertilizers and insecticides used on commercially grown produce. Good health, they said, could only be achieved by eating organically grown food.

Another new industry emerged. Health food stores and organic farms began to prosper. "Organic" fertilizers, vitamins, soap and foods were put on the market. Some people did become more health conscious, but the majority continued on the yummy-tasting path of unwholesome nutrition. Most of us woke up with a bang in the seventies when we were confronted with hard-core facts and unshakable evidence of the rampage of heart disease and cancer among Americans. We did decide to listen, take heed and change our ways once the medical profession took charge as our nutritional guide. We were warned that we were vitamin deficient because our food was nutritionally depleted. What we needed were more vitamins in pill form to supplement our daily food. This advice proved to be an enormous boost for vitamin manufacturers, pharmacies and health-food stores. Americans began an expensive daily intake of vitamins A, B, C, D, E, F, B+, B6, and B12, as well as extra iron, phosphorous, magnesium and potassium.

Salt, thought at one time to stabilize our iodine level, was declared the new enemy. Sugar, too, was held responsible for causing or aggravating diseases. Artificial sweeteners, under attack at various times, became popular again. The sugar substitute was pronounced as the solution to our national sweet tooth. It was proclaimed as nonharmful for diabetics, safe for heart patients, and best of all, as noncaloric and a way to avoid tooth decay.

In the seventies, the cholesterol scare made a significant impact on our daily diet. We were told, this time, that it was cholesterol that was killing us. The American Heart Association issued scientific statistics showing that cholesterol was clogging our arteries, causing arteriosclerosis, and contributing to cardiovascular and circulatory disease. Advertising pitches now denounced all saturated fats as dangerous and hailed the virtues of polyunsaturates. An alarmed public learned everything about saturation ratios and how to cook with polyunsaturated fats. Margarine, which until that time was considered the most lowly of fats, became our most popular polyunsaturated, "highly nutritional" fat product. A new money making industry of low-fat products arose. We began eating synthetics and eliminating such pure and valuable foods as eggs, butter and whole milk. Nonfat or low-fat products cornered the market, and Americans grabbed any packaged food labeled low in cholesterol. The cholesterol panic has now reached explosive proportions. Most whole milk products, such as yogurt and cottage cheese have disappeared from the shelves of supermarkets, and we are literally being forced to buy fat-free or synthetic dairy products. The dangers of cholesterol intake seem to be monitored constantly and consistently. The latest findings have added decaffeinated coffee to the list of no-no's.

Fiber, formerly called roughage, got a tremendous boost in the eighties when President Reagan's colon cancer was diagnosed. Fiber was hailed as a miracle cure. When we were informed that a lack of fiber in our diets was largely responsible for constipation, hemorrhoids and obesity—along with cancer, heart disease and diabetes—supermarket shelves filled with high-fiber products. Drugstores displayed an enormous variety of tablets and other fibrous supplements to soften the stool, stimulate the intestines and reduce weight.

A recent source of inspiration for new books and financial gain was the calcium craze. Calcium made the cover of *Newsweek* as the vitamin of the year. We are now supposedly in great danger of every conceivable disease, from gum infections to osteoporosis, unless we supplement our diets with manufactured calcium or dolomite in pill and powder form. TUMS, otherwise known as an aid to fast relief from heartburn and acid stomach, is recommended by physicians as an excellent source of calcium. As a result, Americans are now swallowing TUMS in enormous amounts. Some people have reported side effects to the excesses: heartburn and acid stomach!

The medical authorities have also decided that obesity along with cholesterol is hazardous to cardiovascular efficiency. Fad diets have mushroomed and it is the rare person who, at one time or another, has not followed some kind of reducing diet. In the United States, we are today obsessively weight conscious, basing standards of beauty, social acceptance and happiness on being skinny, with nary a bulge. Our concern borders on hysteria, and excess weight gain may incite mental anguish, depression and frustration. Paradoxically, we frequently counteract these emotions by eating ourselves into a mountain, adding guilt with every bite, and berating ourselves for lack of willpower. Invariably when we decide to lose weight, we go on whatever reducing plan promises the fastest results.

Millions of dollars are spent on diet pills and even more on so-called meal replacements. The first liquid meals appeared quite a few years ago, but were forced off the shelves when a number of deaths were attributed to them. Sometime later, meal substitutes were produced in powder form and hailed as a nationwide diet aid. Today they are available in either liquid or powder form and are heavily fortified with vitamins and minerals. All promise to be highly nutritious and nourishing, as well as the fastest and most efficient method for shedding pounds. You can buy them in bottles or cans (by the case, if you like) for exorbitant prices. They are often endorsed and acclaimed by superstars in the entertainment field, further encouraging their consumption. The product is usually chocolate or vanilla flavored to disguise the vile taste produced by its equally vile ingredients. The reality is that while they may be as effective for losing weight quickly as any other artificial reducing aid, meal replacements are ineffective for keeping the weight off and potentially more damaging to health than overeating.

Where do we stand at present with nutrition? Are we better off than we were at the beginning of the century when we were ignorant about vitamins and nutritional values and ate what we liked in order to be full? We have definitely made an effort to improve the quality of our nutrition. With the support of Ralph Nader and other enlightened consumer advocates, we have demanded the removal of harmful chemicals from our soil and food products. We have forced the FDA to halt the spraying of field produce with DDT and fluorocarbons, and to ban proven carcinogenic food additives, such as Red Dye #2. We have fought for a reduction in the use of preservative nitrites and we have managed to stop the use of DES to fatten cattle. All of these substances which we consumed for years are, according to current research, lethal to humans. We have forced the manufacturers of processed food to upgrade their nutritional standards and to list their ingredients, so those who purchase prepared products have the option to know exactly what they're getting. Our consumption of red meat is reduced; we eat more poultry and fish. We have also changed our cocktail habits, substituting wine and club soda as aperitifs. We can order decaffeinated coffee and tea in most restaurants. Salad bars have become prominent in many eateries and grocery stores. Whole wheat bread and crackers are now available all over the United States.

Many schools and teachers have cooperated to improve our children's lunches, and many educational districts have voted to remove vending machines in order to eliminate access to candy, ice cream, gum and sodas during school hours. Health food stores are everywhere. We have access to cooperative markets for fresh produce and small farms that can supply us with organically fed poultry and beef. We have come a long way and are now able to eat healthfully and nutritionally if we so choose.

Unfortunately, despite these gains and an increased health consciousness, the greater part of the American population is still eating foods hazardous to their health. Most people today are primarily concerned with feeding themselves cheaply and quickly. Shopping carts are full of processed products: packaged cereals, breads, potato chips, cakes and cookies, frozen dinners, ice cream and canned convenience food. Housewives clip coupons from newspapers, buying products because they are on sale rather than because they're healthful. Even careful consumers are misled by product labeling. They may believe that a product saying "fat free," "diet lite," and "all natural" is really wholesome and nutritious, when it loaded with additives.

The fast food industries are sweeping our nation and other nations as well, because they promise to feed us quickly, cheaply, and—due to the power of advertisement slogans— "nutritionally" as well. Many people, especially our youth, consider a hamburger, French fries, and a Coke a good meal. They seem unaware that the standard hamburger patty is composed of only a small portion of beef, generally imported from other countries, that is cheap, lean, and tough. The other ingredients are domestic fat to make the meat chewable, and soybean flour and other fillers. The skinny patty is the least part of the meal. What fills you up are the white buns, catsup, relish, pickles, potatoes deep-fried in rancid oil, and cola drinks. The commercial hamburger and other "good eatin'" of deep-fried chicken, hot dogs, and similar inferior foods is leading the way to circulatory and intestinal diseases and general deterioration of good health.

People who choose to eat wholesome, natural food believe "You are what you eat." Careful eaters regard bodies as miracles of nature that must be thoughtfully tended. They understand the interconnection between body, mind and spirit. They feed themselves nutritionally because they know that the food chain is their lifeline. Those who are health oriented use their common sense to make choices for themselves, rather than letting outside influences determine what should go into their bodies and what should not. It is not necessary to be fanatic about food, but we must be attentive and concerned so as not to gamble with our health and well-being. Every person can develop and employ good nutritional principles.

Guidelines for Common Sense Nutrition

First and foremost we must realize that food can be beneficial or detrimental, and the intake of so-called good items can never compensate for harmful ones. It is more important to be concerned about what *not* to eat than what to eat, just as it is preferable to stay healthy rather than be ill or run-down.

Eat Natural Foods

Food should be eaten in its natural condition in order to be of greatest benefit to our systems. To subject a human body to foreign substances does not make good sense. Natural foods are those that grow in nature in plant or animal form and are eaten either raw or cooked. They are not processed or canned nor do they come in hermetically sealed plastic packaging or in pill, tablet or powder form. Labels describing contents and ingredients are not necessary. You can recognize what natural foods are just by looking at them. Natural foods spoil, decay and get rancid or stale. In other words, no preservatives are added. Natural foods contain all the vitamins that are required for a healthful existence.

Natural food eating does not need to stand for deprivation. To eat for health only will invariably make Jack a dull boy. Natural foods can turn into exciting meals, presenting a whole new approach to gourmet cooking. Food must please the palate in order for one to maintain good eating habits.

Over-zealous advocates of natural cooking condemn all salts and fats. Current medical and general public opinion, as well, consider salt intake to be hazardous to your health. Yet, salt is not really damaging to the average person, unless one suffers from a congestive heart condition or a specific type of hypertension. It must, of course, be used sparingly, as well as other salty condiments like mayonnaise or mustard. Salads should be the mainstay of everyone's diet, but in order to be and stay exciting, they do need a dash of salt and a sprinkling of fine oil, such as olive, walnut or sesame. (A few drops of vinegar or lemon, of course, and a shake of pepper are also essential for good taste. As long as we're on this subject, please stay away from all commercial salad dressings!) Try to disregard the cholesterol fanatics as well! A tablespoon of oil per day is necessary for your digestion, skin quality and general health.

Steamed vegetables are good to eat on a daily basis—but add a little butter (and salt) and they become even better. It is true that butter is high in cholesterol content and has many calories, which dictates that it should be used in moderation. But it is a pure product and can never be replaced by margarine which is a synthetic substitute of inferior oils, water and diglycerides that deserves to be shunned from the kitchen. Corn and sunflower oils are good for cooking and light frying, but avoid deep frying of food in any kind of fat.

Herbs and exotic spices are essential for any cuisine to emphasize the natural flavors of food. Dill, parsley, chervil, chives, sage, marjoram, caraway seeds, thyme, rosemary and oregano are some, as well as ground or hot pepper, onions, garlic, curry and tumeric. Use whatever amount pleases you, although they may not all agree with your particular digestive system. Lemons act as a wonderful cleansing agent for the entire system. Squeeze them liberally on fish, cooked vegetables, and all compatible foods.

What about the nemesis of health faddists, nutritional counselors and physicians: alcohol, coffee and tea? Hard liquors such as scotch, whiskey and mixed cocktails are harmful to the system, but a fine glass of wine (shop around for wine that is free from sulphates) and a good beer (not canned though) can be uplifting and add festivity to a lovely dinner. Enjoyed occasionally, these beverages enhance any meal. There is certainly caffeine in coffee and tannic acid along with caffeine in tea. Again the key word is moderation. Colas and sodas and chocolate drinks contain as much or more caffeine than coffee. Instant coffee and tea are processed chemically and contain carcinogenic additives. The same used to be the case with decaffeinated coffees but now most are water-processed, and when they are filter-dripped can be as delicious as the real brew. The addition of cream, sugar or artificial sweeteners to coffee and tea compound toxic potential. The indication of a true gourmet is the ability to enjoy a black, sugarless cup of coffee or an expresso with lemon peel without other accompaniment or hint of dessert.

Be Selective About Organic Products

The only way to be positive that you are getting organically grown food is to grow it in your own backyard or buy it directly from a farm where you can trust the farmer. Try to buy your unpackaged grains and cereals, nuts and dried fruits, nut or apple butter, and unprocessed honey in a health food store. But you can purchase fresher and certainly cheaper produce from neighborhood vegetable stores. Avoid supermarkets where fruits and vegetables are apt to ripen in their shipping cases. Investigate community cooperatives and farmers' markets for the best and freshest buys. But make sure that you wash your fruits and vegetables thoroughly, regardless of where you buy them. Some fruits and vegetables need to be peeled (cucumbers, for instance), because their skin is heavily waxed. Don't, however, be a fanatic. While you should make an effort to eat organically grown food, be aware that moderate chemical treatment may be necessary to eliminate parasites and other disease causing organisms from our food supply.

Eat Seasonal Foods

Nature provides us with seasonable foods to maintain our health in each individual season and to get us ready for the next one. We should trust her wisdom. To perpetuate good health we should eat food at its ripest, freshest state. At this point it is full of natural vitamins and nutritional value. We should, in season, stuff ourselves with cherries, plums and peaches and eat all the cobs of fresh corn we can hold. This is how people feed themselves in the rest of the world where their food is obtainable only where and when it grows seasonally. At the peak of ripeness it is eaten in abundance and sometimes preserved in its natural juices for winter storage.

Americans, on the other hand, have strange eating habits. We love tomatoes and eat them all year round, even though they are tasteless, artificially ripened, nutritionally useless and expensive in the winter. We also eat wilted lettuce off season as well as carrots and other vegetables that have been stored in deep freeze. Somehow we even manage to serve canned peas and frozen stringbeans in summer when they are best fresh. By eating fresh, seasonal foods, we increase the nutritional value of our food as well as our eating pleasure.

Moderate Your Meat Intake

We have been misled into believing that large amounts of protein are essential to a good diet and that we must eat large quantities of meat to fulfill our daily protein requirement. It has been documented that the average American eats twice the protein that his body can use. Since protein is not stored by our bodies, whatever is not used is wasted. Athletes, whose training program used to call for huge amounts of meat, have recently switched to carbohydrates, vegetables and fruits instead. This apparently allows them to perform better, feel better and have more energy. You will feel the same benefit from reducing your meat intake as these athletes.

Substitute for meat other protein sources. There is actually as much protein contained in fish, eggs and cheese as there is in meat. Nuts and legumes—dried beans, peas and lentils— are perhaps the finest source of protein. Protein is found in every living food, especially in all green leafy vegetables. Interestingly, nutritional studies have revealed that when inhabitants of nations which experienced meat shortages during World War II were forced to supplement their diets with other protein foods, they were generally healthier than during their meat-eating years.

Vitamins

Perversely, we Americans create vitamin deficiencies by eating processed food and then take artificial vitamins to alleviate our self-made deprivation. Our actions only add to the already monumental income of the vitamin industry, which is selling us products that are both costly and nonessential. Organic and artificial vitamins are derived from natural foods. The hull of rice, wheat germ and bran that is discarded by the miller is sold to the vitamin manufacturer. We are in the ironic position of buying back the original, nutritious food product, second or third hand, in concentrated capsule form. In earlier periods, it was possible to live "by bread alone," because all the natural nutritional value was left in the food where it belonged.

While it is true that processed and chemically produced foods have been stripped of much of their food value, the vitamin industry has exaggerated for its own benefit the need for supplemental vitamins. Actually, we need only minuscule amounts of vitamins to stay well. One stalk of broccoli is sufficient for daily vitamin A content. A tablespoon of oil provides you with all necessary vitamin E. A spinach leaf gives you ample vitamin B, and one fruit per day supplies your full need for vitamin C.

There is a legitimate place for vitamins, just as there is for drugs, in the treatment of certain diseases. Vitamin supplements are excellent therapy for restoring tissue damage for burn victims. Alcoholics, drug addicts, and people with digestive diseases who can't absorb their foods may suffer from vitamin depletion. Additional vitamins may also be indicated in cases of extreme fatigue, during pregnancy, in drastic instances of metabolic body changes, and whenever fresh produce is not available.

But vitamins are drugs and they may be harmful when used indiscriminately. It is a widely believed fallacy that overdosing is safe because all vitamins are water soluble and excess amounts will pass through the bloodstream. Our bodies do excrete excess amounts of some vitamins, but most are stored in body fat and can accumulate significantly. Many people, furthermore, are allergic to vitamins, although they may be unaware of the condition. No one — pharmacist, health food store proprietor, holistic practitioner, or accredited physician — has the knowledge to prescribe vitamins for your individual requirements. Everything is hit-or-miss guesswork, because it is scientifically impossible to determine how much of which vitamin a certain body needs.

It is illogical to presume, for example, that a woman who weighs 100 pounds requires the same amount of supplements as a 200 pound man. Also, our physical systems undergo constant biological, biochemical, and biorhythmic changes in response to our hormonal balances, menstrual cycles, and mental condition. Even though a supplement is indicated today, it may be superfluous tomorrow. Some physicians advocate blood, urine or hair testing to determine vitamin deficiencies, but will admit that none of these tests are conclusive. Many chiropractors and holistic experts employ muscle testing, as part of applied kinesiology, to determine which vitamins are needed. These techniques certainly cannot harm you, if you have the time and money to investigate. But they are not guaranteed. If you eat good food, exercise daily, breathe correctly and deeply, and think good thoughts, you will not need supplementary vitamins to assure your good health. You will never even catch a cold.

Eat Only When You Are Hungry

Some people can go without food all day and require only one large meal. Others may have hypoglycemia or diabetic predispositions and become nervous and upset when their blood sugar level fluctuates. They need to eat more often and in smaller quantities. Eat as your stomach, not the clock, commands. There is no reason to stick to a three-meal routine when you are comfortable eating only two. Many people, especially Europeans, prefer to eat a large meal at noon and a light one at night. They recognize that going to sleep on a full stomach can cause insomnia, indigestion, constipation and obesity.

Many working people eat breakfast out of habit rather than according to appetite. They have a Danish or doughnut when it is coffee break time and eat lunch when it is lunch time, simply because the clock says they should. But other people are getting smarter. They're learning to eat only when their body says they should. They take an apple or yogurt to work and use their lunch time to walk, run or take an exercise class. On the other hand, you don't want to let yourself get to the point of such extreme hunger that you'll wolf down your food ravenously. A healthy appetite means enjoying food when you are hungry and not devouring large quantities.

Drink Only When You Are Thirsty

Water is your finest beverage but the accepted rule of drinking eight glasses per day is without scientific foundation. Tap water today is contaminated in many areas of the country and the addition of fluoride, a powerful toxin, does not make it a desirable drink. Plutonium has penetrated the New York City water supply, which used to be one of the purest. Attach a filtering system to your faucet or try to drink bottled water in all areas of questionable water purity. Also avoid drinking iced water, especially as an accompaniment to meals. Ice produces a shock when it touches your skin. Imagine then how it can jolt your internal organs when it is gulped down. It is not good to drink large quantities of beverages with meals, either. Instead, try slowly sipping a glass of dry wine as you eat. It is less caloric, a more natural beverage than sweet soda drinks, and can be an aid to digestion.

I can think of no other country in the world where people, especially the young, flood their systems with so many soda drinks and juices. (The barter in empty soda cans has turned into a flourishing enterprise for the unemployed all through the U.S.) All canned and bottled drinks are devoid of nutriments, bloating, and harmful to the system, regardless of whether they are sugared or sugarless (which means artificially sweetened). All are chockful of chemicals; avoid them.

Don't Overeat

Most of us eat too much and indiscriminately. We clean our plates because we have been taught to do so, and stop eating only when we are completely stuffed. Overloading the digestive system is perhaps more detrimental to our health than anything else. Also, it is unthinkable for some Americans to finish a meal without dessert, and they literally "make room" for it. Youngsters need food for growth, but it stands to reason that a body which is no longer growing does not need as much food. If you are over thirty-five and less physically active, you will burn fewer calories than when you were young. All surplus food will be carried around as fat by older, more sedentary adults. The most healthful change in eating habits you can make is to learn to stop eating before you are completely full.

Avoid Dieting

Whatever you do, don't "go" on a diet. The very word, except when correctly applied to everyday sustenance, is self-defeating. Most people go on a diet only to get off it again. All fad diets work because one can lose weight on any monotonous eating routine, whether it's all fruit, all protein, all carbohydrates, or liquid meals. Each one produces a weight loss but the effects last only a short time. As soon as the individual returns to his usual eating habits the weight reappears, often in greater excess. No pill or extreme diet produces permanent results because unnatural forms of eating are eventually rejected by our mental and physical system. Every disciplinary eating regimen leads to frustration if it fails to please the palate. People who have no weight problems love vegetables, salads and fruits. Their idea of fun is to chew on a raw carrot. Those who are overweight love manufactured sweets along with heavy, spicy food.

One can lose weight and keep it off without causing physical or mental anguish. First must come the decision that you really want to be slim, not because everyone says that you should be, but because you would rather look good in your clothes than eat chocolate cake. You can't have both. You should also realize that drastic weight fluctuation damages your system and causes premature sagging and wrinkling of your skin. Rather than going up and down in weight, it may be more healthful for you to stay chubby. Your best insurance in reaching a healthy old age is to stabilize your weight, never gaining or losing more than five pounds.

Once you have made up your mind, accept the fact that you can only lose weight on a permanent basis if you commit yourself to daily exercise. This may be contrary to the opinions of some diet doctors and diet books. They may acknowledge the need for exercise but only as an adjunct to the prescribed dietary regimen. But in fact, exercise is the primary requirement for maintaining normal weight.

If you can do nothing else, start out with one mile of slow walking and gradually increase the speed and the distance. When you are lighter and more energetic, go on to race-walking or bicycling. Buy yourself a rebounder for rainy days. Try Yoga exercises, together with breathing, meditation and relaxation. Either follow this book or take lessons. If that is not your cup of tea, find an exercise program that pleases you. You could join a group in which overweight people discuss their individual problems. But don't follow their diets or adhere to their lack of exercise.

Realize that you may be a carbohydrate junkie and, like an alcoholic or a nicotine addict who can never take a drink or smoke a cigarette, you cannot cope with sweets and starches. Sugar is your nemesis, and artificial sweeteners do *not* make you thin and are dangerous to your health to boot. On the other hand, also forget about calorie counting. Do not embark on a diet of lettuce leaves, carrots, celery, melba toast and other dull foods. Boring deprivation will cause you to be overwhelmed by self-pity and revert to your old eating habits. Think of yourself as a person who can eat normally but is going to change eating patterns. You are going to substitute delicious nonfattening, nutritious food for fattening, unhealthy food and you won't be deprived or hungry. With the money that you used to spend on junk foods, treat yourself to the most exquisite fruits, like strawberries, pineapple, mangoes, kiwis and bananas, which are also most filling.

You will eat the most attractive salads and only eat those vegetables that you like, and you will learn to love eating everything that swims. Always be sure to have snacks around so that you don't get into trouble. Stock up on the good kind: sunflower seeds, fruits, vegetables, cold boiled chicken, rice cakes or bread sticks, and European crisp breads that are free from additives and taste yummy even without butter. Pamper yourself, praise yourself, love yourself and don't berate yourself for your lack of willpower. If you take an occasional misstep, dust yourself off and get back on the horse.

Eat For Pleasure

In addition to being a basic drive, eating can be one of our greatest pleasures. We have made great strides during the last decade to improve our cuisine, but we still have a long way to go to master the fine art of dining. The French are of course the acclaimed experts on *haute cuisine,* as are most Europeans. Yet we don't need to cook in the heavily sauced, Continental manner with lots of butter and cream in order to enjoy gourmet meals. It is possible to adapt gourmet cooking methods to produce meals that are natural, light and flavorful. A meal, especially dinner, can represent a break in the routine, an enjoyable interlude with family or friends and a treat to the senses. It should be the most pleasant time of the day, not an interruption to a television program or a shove-and-gulp routine at a fast food emporium.

Try to pay more attention to your surroundings. Never eat standing up or at your desk while talking on the phone, no matter how great your hurry. At dinner time make the effort to eat at an attractively set table, even if it is in the kitchen. Use your good dishes and silver and fine glasses. You are as deserving as the most revered guest. Treat yourself well, especially if you live alone. Nothing is more depressing than eating out of a carton or on paper or plastic dishes. With all the instant food crowding supermarket shelves it seems comprehensible that our future food may come in pill form; breakfast, lunch and dinner will be three quick swallows! I sincerely hope that we can forestall this appalling prospect by reviving the joy of gracious dining.

Learn to Eat Slowly

Do you know who eats slowly? People who are thin.

Overweight people often gulp their food, wash it down with fluids, or eat on the run. But those who take the time to savor each bite find they eat less and enjoy their food more. Also, chewing slowly is the answer to most digestive troubles. The healthy stomach of a normal person can cope with almost any food if it has been thoroughly chewed.

Get Into the Raw Juice Habit

Instead of filling up on canned and processed fruit juices, look into the therapeutic values of freshly squeezed juices. It is time consuming to squeeze vegetables by hand and a juicer is expensive. But for those who think they need to supplement their diet with artificial vitamins, a juicer is a far superior investment. In their concentrated form raw juices are excellent for rebuilding and maintaining health. Carrot juice, one of the richest sources of vitamin A, is frequently called a miracle juice for the cure and prevention of colds, kidney and bladder infections, and helps to strengthen the eyes. However, excess ingestion of carrot juice can lead to carotene poisoning, just as anything that is carried to excess can be harmful.

Fast Periodically

It makes good sense to cleanse the inside of your body occasionally and rest the digestive organs, which work constantly. If you set aside one day per month when you can rest at home, and rest your inner system as well, you will feel wonderfully light for the remainder of the week. Drink water with lemon or fresh vegetable juice or enjoy vegetable broth. You may be hungry at first but your hunger pangs will subside. Try to go through the day without eating, but if you are too uncomfortable by evening eat a vegetable or baked potato or another light meal. During illness make it a point to fast.

Fasting is also a most effective way of reducing. On a low-calorie, three-meals-a-day diet, for instance, you will find yourself suffering hunger from one skinny meal to the next. If you stop eating completely, you will experience hunger pangs for only one day. On the second day you will feel great, and even better on ensuing days. Best of all, the pounds will roll off. Drink only when thirsty and avoid coffee, tea and all toxins. You can work and exercise without feeling weak, nor will you starve. The more weight you have to lose the longer you can keep fasting. A prolonged fast, however, should not be undertaken without medical supervision.

Children's Nutrition

Good eating habits can be started at any time to improve everyone's life but are, of course, most beneficial when established during childhood. Mother's milk is the foundation for a healthy child and babies should be breast fed whenever possible. If breast feeding is not possible, a good substitute can be found in soy milk since many babies are allergic to cow's milk, and most pre-mixed formulas contain artificial ingredients.

Commercial baby foods are processed with additives like sodium and refined sugar which don't belong in a baby's sensitive system. Until it was banned even MSG was put into baby foods. If you love your baby, mash bananas and other fruits for him, also grate apples and puree fresh vegetables. Babies love squash, sweet potatoes and yams. When he toddles and has only three teeth let him eat what you eat, provided you eat good food. As he gets older, get him accustomed to chewing on carrots and hard bread crusts for roughage and strong teeth. Your child does not need cookies, cupcakes, ice cream, sugared cereals, candy, gum or soda drinks except on special occasions. Products labeled sugar-free should definitely be avoided. Sugar-free stands for artificially sweetened and health hazardous.

If you are really concerned with your child's health refuse to believe that anything in a can, box or plastic container is healthful and nutritious. Always keep fresh fruit handy or dried fruits like raisins and apricots. Purchase sunflower seeds, unsalted nuts and fresh nuts for your family to crack. Do your child a favor and don't support the fast-food restaurants, drive-ins and take-outs. For special family outings habituate restaurants where delicious, healthy food is available. In Chinese restaurants ask for food without MSG. A good parent is one who is able to say "no" firmly when the kids demand hot dogs, candy and junk food because the detrimental effects of these foods are recognized. Good parents know that no amount of so-called right foods can counteract the damage done by wrong foods.

We are under the misconception that our children's good health depends upon drinking lots of milk and orange juice. Besides restoring the blood sugar level that is lost during sleep, orange juice is of little value when it is canned, frozen or comes in plastic containers. In these forms it is depleted of natural nutriments and augmented with artificial vitamins. Freshly squeezed orange juice does contain all natural vitamins, but it also has a lot of natural sugar and nobody needs that many

vitamins or sugar in one glass. One orange eaten whole, preferably with some of the skin and pulp, fulfills our vitamin
requirements to the brim.

As for milk drinking, Americans tend to think that if children drink three glasses of milk a day they will be healthy.
Milk is high in protein, minerals and vitamins and is easily
digestible for the average child, but does not alone provide
total health. Moreover, drinking milk in excess may not be
good for everyone. In some countries, goat or yak milk is considered superior to cow's milk. And many current theorists
uphold that only mother's milk is the proper nourishment for
a child.

Meal Suggestions

Bear in mind that the following suggestions are intended
for the average, sedentary adult with normal body proportions
who wishes to stay slim. Children need to eat differently and
so do people wth large physiques or specific health needs. It is
understood that an athlete or hard-working laborer who burns
up a great number of calories during the day requires additional, possibly different foods.

Breakfast

Right now, the first thing in the morning, begin relying
on the good judgment of your own body instead of what people
say you must do. Forget that you *must* have a big breakfast.
Never eat when you don't feel like eating or force your children to do so. Some people enjoy a large breakfast, especially
on weekends, while others shudder at the thought. If you are
not hungry, drink a glass of water or another beverage, have a
piece of fruit, or skip breakfast altogether. You will feel less
hungry at lunch time. If you have a weight problem get used
to eating nothing but fruit until lunch time. Fruits retain their
full vitamin content and are more easily digested and less fattening when they are eaten as a separate meal. Cooked cereals
like oatmeal, Wheatina, Cream of Wheat, rice or grits are
filling and nutritious, even when cooked in water. Sweeten them
with a little honey, fruit or pure fruit juice.

At present, the cereal industry would have you believe that
they hold the monopoly on keeping you disease free. They
advertise products like oat bran that will lower your choles-

terol, prevent cancer and insure you a long life. If you like cold cereal, eat it by all means. But select the whole wheat, unsweetened product or make your own granola. Muesli, imported from Switzerland, contains wheat germ, oats, millet flakes, fruit and no storage preservative. Skip french toast made from white bread drenched in syrup. Make pancakes and waffles from wheat flour. Have one egg, not two or three, and definitely omit bacon and sausage. Eggs don't need to be fried, scrambled or otherwise disguised. It is deliciously civilized to spoon a soft or medium-boiled egg from the top of a china eggcup.

If you cannot do without toast, shop for a bread that lists "stone ground whole wheat flour" with its contents. Even better, eat a slice of crusted, freshly baked wheat, rye or pumper-nickel bread, easily available in good bakeries. Don't put butter or margarine on your bread; it is a fattening combination. Instead try cottage cheese or natural apple, plum or nut butter as a spread. These will also satisfy your craving for something sweet. Drink your beverage after the meal. There is no reason that you need to limit yourself to the traditional breakfast foods of this country. You may feel like eating left-over chicken, kippers or noodles. Japanese eat soup for their morn-ing meal. Kibbutz members in Israel breakfast on salads, olives and white cheese. They seem to have all the energy they need to drive tractors and plow the fields.

Lunch

If you had a big breakfast go easy on lunch. Unless it's your first meal of the day, skip it altogether or just have a piece of fruit. But don't do this if it means you'll be ravenous by supper time. If you have to eat twice as much at dinner because you omitted lunch, you are doubly defeating your purpose.

Lunch can present a problem for working people who wish to eat wholesomely. The sandwich, hamburger and hot dog on a bun are three American institutions that everyone could do without. Bread, regardless of its variety, is not only fattening but is also a superfluous starch that should be eaten in small quantities. Avoid sandwiches if you can or try whole wheat pita or imported rye-crisps instead of standard breads. Cross off luncheon meats, sausage and ham from your shop-ping list. While you are at it, eliminate delicatessen goodies as well. How can you give up bagels, cream cheese and lox (smoked salmon)? Don't, but limit these to rare occasions.

Cottage cheese or feta cheese are good sandwich fillings but stay away from creamy and processed cheeses. Yogurt is great for lunch, and so is a beautiful salad.

Try to wean yourself away from our most popular lunchtime staple, tuna fish. Canned fish are lifeless vittles. If you must eat tuna fish, pour off the oil and go easy on the mayo. Cold chicken or fish are good substitutes for tuna. So is a hardboiled egg, unless you had one for breakfast. Excellent sandwich fillings can be made from ripe tomatoes, sprouts and avocados. Avocados are a fabulous food and contain almost every nutrient that is needed by your system. Avocados are not fattening when eaten separately, rather than as part of the meal.

When eating lunch at a restaurant find an appetizing salad of greens, spinach or vegetables, an omelet or piece of fish if you are involved in executive dining. Salad bars present the alternative to eating junk food, but the edibles are often of questionable freshness. Cases of botulin poisoning have been traced to salad bars. One can't be too particular with restaurant food, but I prefer to wash my own salad greens if I have the choice. Also the creamy dressings that come with the salad bars are high in calories and loaded with additives. Drink your favorite herb tea, decaffeinated coffee or Perrier before or after, but not with, your lunch.

Dinner

It's a good idea, especially for the weight watcher, to have a beverage before dinner; fresh vegetable juice, vegetable broth or plain club soda. If you go out to dinner or are at a party, sip your dinner wine as an aperitif or have a wine spritzer. Try artichoke vinaigrette as the first course at a restaurant as well as at home. You could also begin with a small cup of soup, unless you choose to have a meal of hearty soup and a big salad. Consomme or plain chicken, vegetable, bean or lentil soups are delicious and nutritious in home-made versions. You can also eat your salad as a first course.

Try to cut down on eating meat, but don't overlook organ meats. Liver, kidneys, brains and sweetbreads are excellent sources of protein, are easy to digest and also inexpensive. If you have poultry, stay away from the skin. It is pure fat, difficult to digest and an enemy of the gall bladder. If fresh fish is not available, substitute frozen fish, which is preferable to hot dogs and TV dinners. Salmon, sole, halibut and swordfish are the most popular fresh fish, though their prices are unaffordable for many. There are lots of other delicious fish varieties — blue fish, trout, mackeral, smelts, catfish, or tilefish — which are just as tasty and inexpensive.

As a result of the cholesterol scare, fish oil capsules are the latest fad in nutritional supplements. Americans who used to balk at downing their weekly ration of cod liver oil are consuming fish oil capsules en masse. It is said that eating more fish reduces heart disease and may prevent arthritis and cancer. But no one has yet determined whether the body can safely absorb megadoses of fish oil in capsules. Eating fish in its natural state is by far the safer and certainly the more tasty way to stave off threatening diseases. Make an effort to avoid all fish and seafood that live in shallow waters and stick to the deep sea or pure stream variety.

Have a salad or cooked vegetables with your meal. Experiment with all the varieties of lettuce and other salad plants, like Boston, bibb, romaine, chicory and radiccio, if you wish to splurge. Iceberg lettuce is the most popular type of lettuce in this country, but it is tasteless and lowest in vitamin content. Anything fresh and green can be used in a salad, even those vegetables we usually cook, such as spinach, cabbage, cauliflower, broccoli, mushrooms, and zucchini. Cube, dice or break endives, radishes, cucumbers, red and green peppers, watercress and avocado into a salad, also red onions, scallions, chives, parsley and fresh dill. Experiment with all the different vegetables that are in season. Steam or cook them in a minimal amount of salted water for only a few minutes, so they remain crunchy. Then drain and add a little butter, parsley, dill or other seasoning. You will never revert to frozen or canned vegetables after experiencing the real thing. Vegetables cooked in a microwave oven are uniformly delicious as well. Steamed in their own juice, they require no other enhancement.

Don't combine potatoes with meat, rice with chicken, or horror of horrors, spaghetti with meatballs. Animal protein and starches are an extremely fattening combination and do not mix well in the stomach. Learn about all the varieties of beans, lentils and other legumes that are available. As complementary proteins they mix beautifully with rice or tortillas and other grains. Investigate the nourishing, protein-rich qualities of tofu and tempeh, and use them to accompany rice and vegetables. The Oriental cuisine is generally healthier and more easily digestible than ours. Experiment with stir frying as an alternative way of cooking. You could build a whole meal around a baked potato, a rice dish like pilaf, a bulgar wheat casserole, or pasta made from wheat flour, spinach or semolina. Combined with a non-starchy vegetable and a salad, these present a nourishing way of eating, even for the weight watcher.

Now we come to dessert, and this course poses the biggest problem. If you can, learn to give it up. If you can't do without, fresh fruit is the best solution. Select seasonable berries, melon, pineapple or a fresh fruit salad. Consider nuts or dried fruits such as raisins, dates, figs, apricots, apples and plums. These will satisfy anyone's sweet tooth but they are high in calories. Better yet, treat yourself to a cappuccino.

Be aware that you are a special person, with special tastes and inclinations. No one can tell you what, how and when to eat. Only you can make those decisions. The same is true for children. A young child will instinctively choose the food that is most suitable for his system. Once you have been conditioned to regular exercise and proper breathing, you will automatically become more aware of your body's needs. You will choose to eat what your body demands and reject the food that may harm it. Some people function best on a vegetarian diet, others feel better when they eat fish, eggs or meat. Don't forget that your body is changing constantly, in both metabolism and age. The foods that felt right to you last year may not feel best for you now. Listen to your body. It is extremely intelligent and will always lead you in the right direction.

The common sense rule for good nutrition is moderation. You need not denounce the foods that you and your family consider delicious because they don't measure up to nutritional standards. Don't ever be a fanatic about food, or anything else for that matter. To be a food fanatic is as unhealthy as being a food junkie. Anyone who faints at the sight of meat or refuses to sample a seven-layer chocolate cake at a party is a killjoy! To consume ice cream, cake, cookies, hot dogs, pizza, colas and cocktails as a daily habit is senseless and detrimental to your health. But there is nothing wrong in having these treats once in a while.

When you do indulge, make an effort to acquire the best piece of chocolate, the most delectable pastry, the finest ice cream. Enjoy and don't feel guilty. Remember that habitual exercise makes up for all dietary trespasses. Your trained body will effortlessly avoid foods that interfere with its optimal performance.

Part Two
Spiritual Awakening

CHAPTER SIX

The Role of Meditation

W e now enter the most profoundly rewarding aspect of our holistic journey: the
expansion of our mental capacities and the
realization of our spiritual potential. We know
that it is possible to bring about significant physical changes by applying common sense techniques. No expensive supplementary therapies are needed. There are no courses
or lectures to attend. No health experts who charge a fee for
leading the way. All that is required is the decision to make
changes and the will to follow through. Once we are headed in
the right direction it is amazing what we can accomplish; even
those in poor physical condition with limited expectations for
success will experience positive changes. By following a program of effective exercise, proper breathing and healthful
nutrition, we can achieve physical fitness in a relatively short
time. As we feel more energetic and healthier, our discipline
takes on new meaning and becomes easier to pursue.

Everything that does not please us can be changed, even
our system of thought. Just as we can make physical changes
in our favor, we can make mental ones as well. Unproductive
and unhealthy thoughts can be brought into our daily consciousness and made to disappear. Just as we acknowledge that
there is no need to be physically ill, we can become aware that
mental unhappiness and sickness are also unnecessary.
Convinced that life doesn't make sense without inner serenity,
we become able to say, "I am happy, I am peaceful."

Everyone wants to be happy and peaceful, but few actually are because we seek happiness in the wrong places in outside events, possessions, and other people. Although we are
programmed to look outside ourselves for contentment, the
truth is that it can only be found within ourselves. Each of us
has had our share of mishaps, but we each view these mishaps

with different states of mind, rather like looking through different lenses. One person may cut his finger, get a Band-Aid and forget about it. Another will suffer and create a major crisis from a minor incident. Individuals who are maimed, deformed or otherwise underprivileged are often able to achieve contentment and fulfillment. Others generate additional handicaps for themselves.

Most people function at peak capacity only when circumstances are favorable — the weather is good, the train is punctual, the boss is jovial, and all the family are well. External conditions can make life pleasant or unpleasant. But, ultimately, our response to external conditions is shaped by our state of mind. Our own thoughts determine whether we feel joy or sorrow, health or illness, hate or love, fear or peace.

Harnessing the mind, however, is extremely difficult. The mind likes variety and constant movement. It is so active that while we are in one place, the mind races forward or back to another place, another time. Nor can we turn our minds off, even during sleep. When we dream our mental powers are often at peak activity. Sometimes we attempt to anesthetize our brains with alcohol or drugs, but the consciousness has not stopped. We may feel it is impossible to calm the turbulence of our thoughts. When this turbulence feels painful and confusing, we often use a belligerent approach, attempting to rationalize, scold or fantasize our problems away. Of course this never works. Most of the time it intensifies the pain and confusion that we want to eliminate. Some people find relief from the turmoil in their minds with psychiatric help, but psychotherapy is usually a lengthy and arduous process. Hypnosis and biofeedback can be helpful. Prayer provides relief for some.

I believe the least complicated way to change and rest the mind is through meditation. Meditation is also the most enjoyable and the least time-consuming of all methods. Meditation is neither mysterious nor occult. It is not a religious, esoteric or glamorous practice. When stripped of all philosophical and psychological contexts, it is simple; to meditate means to let go of all thoughts. It is not to contemplate but to un-think. Meditation is mental relaxation, crucial for our sense of well-being.

The mind is like a giant computer, a storehouse of factual information. Each experience, thought and dream is recorded from the time of birth to the present moment. The mind is prepared to accept an endless stream of input. Crowded in with daydreams and speculations about the future are guilt and regrets about the past. As there is no release valve to empty the contents, our mind is neither cleaned nor aired. Not surprisingly it is often in poor health.

Modern medical and psychiatric practitioners are keenly aware that mind relaxation, in addition to sleep, is essential for both physical and psychological fitness. No longer do they insist that the cure for stress is to be found in ordinary, relaxing activities such as catnaps, gardening or sitting quietly with our feet up. They have conceded that the regular practice of deep mind relaxation can strengthen the immune system, relieve pain, lower blood pressure and promote healing. Heart and breath rates can also be slowed. Research has demonstrated that meditation may help ward off disease by making people less susceptible to viruses as well as heart attacks.

Psychiatry has taught us that it is usually the quality of thoughts that causes mental illness. The way we see ourselves in relation to the rest of the world strongly influences our happiness and well-being. Some of our thoughts are positive, full of purpose and meaning, but the majority are ineffectual and trivial. Running through the mind are also thoughts of greed, envy and malice, as well as worry, grief and fear. These thoughts are harmful to no one but ourselves, they are like poison to the system, causing us sickness and unhappiness.

Ancient man understood the biological impact of mind relaxation. Throughout time sages have advocated setting aside time to arrest mental activity so that the body and mind could be refreshed. This practice enabled man to cope more efficiently with the challenges of daily tasks in often hostile environments. Places of worship were built so that individuals could sit in solitude, discovering the meaning of life in the innermost depths of the self. Sanctuaries, such as pagodas, altars, shrines, mosques and temples, still exist all over the world for quiet reflection and meditation. Meditation is not to be confused with prayer. To pray means to implore something from someone. This can have healing benefits as well, but meditation specifically means to turn within, to find the meaning of life in the interior landscape, not in outside forces.

Various meditation techniques exist, but the goal is the same: to achieve God realization and God-consciousness. The apex of meditation is the state of unity with cosmic consciousness, where one's body and ordinary mind are transcended so that the spirit becomes all. The soul is liberated and released from the world of things as they seem. The physical body no longer exists. Body, mind and spirit are united with infinity.

Earlier in this century those who meditated were labeled peculiar. But in recent years the practice has been revived as Transcendental Meditation, TM, and become a fashionable pastime. One cartoon caption read, "I'll tell you my mantra, if you'll tell me yours." TM is a structured mind relaxation based on Mantra concentration. In essence, it is an ancient and infinitesimal part of Yoga meditation.

TM was a revelation to those who had never taken the time to sit quietly and do nothing. Extremely tense people found an immediate release from stress. Meditators reported lowered blood pressure, reduced metabolic and heart rates, and decreased anxiety and tension. They achieved better performance in general, with higher levels of energy, productivity and well-being. Often it worked wonders where psychiatry and tranquilizers failed. Purely as a mind relaxation, it is very helpful and easily adaptable to a Western lifestyle. I know quite a few people who have greatly benefited by its practice and used it as a stepping stone to spiritual advancement. But although it is still taught, TM has lost much of its popularity because it was initiated as a money-making enterprise, pitched to fad-conscious achievers. As such it has been superseded by similar techniques under different names. TM has been successful because it is uncomplicated. But there is no depth to it philosophically, nor is there anything from which to build and develop. It is like a prefabricated house with no foundation. The emphasis on mental aspects ignores the physical body.

A holistic lifestyle provides a sturdy foundation, for body and mind are regarded as a single entity in a continuous state of interaction. TM and similar techniques can bring about temporary changes, but the application of holism is insurance for a lifetime of physical and mental health. If we approach meditation via the practice of physical principles, we build a natural and meaningful road to follow. A person with a strong, healthy body voluntarily seeks insight. When a body is in a maximum state of health and perfectly attuned, meditation is always easier. When people prepare their bodies and inadvertently their minds through exercise, breathing and good nutrition, they make a natural transition into the higher aspects of the mind. When we reach a meditative state by following the holistic path, it is a profound experience which can become an integral part of our life structure.

Meditation cannot be forced, it has to come about naturally. It should be pursued because there is a will, a need or a desire. Like any lifelong self-discipline, meditation works only if it is pleasurable. It may be a regimented mental practice, but to establish it as an integral aspect of daily life we must welcome it, giving it preference over some other activities. Eventually meditation becomes such a rich part of our experience that we feel a void if we miss it for a single day.

There are many schools of thought in philosophy, psychology and science about how many levels of consciousness exist and what precisely these are. I find it useful to talk about three levels: the conscious, the subconscious, and the superconscious mind. The conscious or everyday mind is usually referred to as the rational mind, the one with which we are most familiar since we believe it to be in charge of our functioning on this earth. Sometimes it is described as intelligence, psyche or ego. This is the mind that copes with the mechanical and technical problems of day-to-day living. It can tell us how to handle our business, how much money we have in the bank, how to cross the street, what to have for dinner and so forth. Yet it only handles a part of our experience and cannot take care of all our problems.

In meditation, we reach the subconscious level of the mind and stay in this state as long as we desire. We all experience this state frequently, though fleetingly, when we watch a good performance, read an interesting book, or daydream. Total absorbance in active sports, such as running, skiing and long-distance swimming can also produce a meditative state. T'ai Chi Chuan is a meditation in motion, and so is the practice of Hatha Yoga when the concentration is focused on the breath. Whenever we involuntarily focus our attention on something apart from day-to-day existence we make contact with this powerful force within us. In the practice of meditation we seek out the subconscious and let the conscious mind take a back seat for awhile. We remain fully conscious but surface thoughts become subdued, less pressing and more refined. By giving the mind a rest from the continuous surface activity we are able to view its thoughts, sort them out, and channel them in the direction we desire. We learn to silence the conscious mind, quieting its endless chatter, and get in touch with our deeper selves. We can gain new insights into ourselves and learn to function more efficiently.

Through diligent practice and earnest motivation it is

possible to achieve the highest level of meditation, Samadhi or Nirvana in Sanskrit, Satori in Japanese. Samadhi is the state of superconsciousness, the greatest bliss. It is the cessation of personal thoughts and desires. This is the supreme union, the merger of body, mind and spirit into one entity. In this state we let go of the apparent self to reach the true self, which is at one with all things in the universe. An ecstatic sensation, this feeling can help us overcome our fears and illuminate our daily existence. Most of us are not ready for superconsciousness, however, as it takes many years of training to reach this state.

The subconscious level can be the desired state to reach in meditation, and can help you achieve a more meaningful sense of your everyday role. With meditation, you can become master of your mind. With that mastery comes the power to choose thoughts that are pleasing and useful. As you work toward this mastery, you will discover that your ability to concentrate increases. You will be able to focus your attention more intensely without being distracted, making it easier to accomplish all the tasks before you. Each person has the capacity for significant purpose and tranquility. This potential can be realized once the powers of the mind are harnessed into beneficial channels. When thought determines action, there is strength to undertake and carry out what we once considered hopeless and impossible. Fears and self-doubt become manageable as we become peaceful and quiet.

How to Practice Meditation

Successful meditation does not depend on how long you practice. Even five minutes of daily practice can bring results. The ascetic meditates for many hours, but half an hour is usually sufficient for our needs. Like Hatha Yoga and other physical disciplines, meditation can be a purely mechanical part of one's daily routine. It is the regularity that produces results. Set aside fifteen minutes in the beginning. Try hard to adhere to that period of time. Have a clock nearby and hold yourself to the full fifteen minutes. Gradually increase the length of time. Eventually you may want to meditate twice each day, but don't exceed thirty minutes per session. When you are on vacation and have more free time, you may want to meditate longer.

The process of meditation is simple, but it is not that easy to master. Your goal is to suspend thinking, eventually clearing your mind of all thought. Try being thoughtless for thirty seconds and you will see how difficult it is. Or attempt to hold on to just one thought and you will discover that you are thinking about ten different things simultaneously. As you begin to practice the technique, thoughts will slip in from all directions to interfere with your meditation. It is best not to struggle against or squelch these intrusive thoughts. Accept them as part of yourself and let them be. The way to practice successful meditation is to acknowledge your everyday thoughts without impatience or judgment. Tell them gently to go away and to come back later. They will eventually abate and finally dissipate.

Meditation can be done anywhere but it is most successful when performed in beautiful surroundings. Nothing is more conducive to meditation than the beauties of nature. Anyone who has meditated on a mountaintop or beside a waterfall will tell you so. Wherever or whenever you meditate, make sure you choose a quiet time and a place where you will not be interrupted. Try to anticipate and deter all possible disturbances. For instance, take the phone off the hook. Silence adds to the quality of your meditation. Complete stillness, however, is not mandatory for meditation. Inner tranquility will compensate for outside noise.

Sit on the floor with crossed legs, or on a chair with feet flat on the floor or wherever you are most comfortable. The Lotus pose is optional for those with flexible knees. Avoid slouching against an overstuffed chair or couch and do not lie down. You want to maintain a straight spine, which is imperative to avoid going to sleep.

It is very helpful to relax the body before meditation. Let your mind concentrate on your head, relaxing the top of the head and the brain. Direct your eyelids to become very heavy as they fall over the eyes. Let all your facial features drop. Release the tension in the back of the neck, the shoulders, the arms and hands. Relax the torso, particularly the muscles in the back and around each vertebra. Deeply relax the abdominal muscles. It is very important to eliminate strain in the abdominal area. Relax the pelvis, the legs and feet. Harmonious breathing is also necessary for successful meditation. After you have relaxed your body continue with about five minutes of deep breathing. Refer to the breathing section of this book for instructions.

The steps to meditation are concentration and contemplation. Before we can empty the mind of all thought we must practice concentration. In this stage you learn to focus on one thought only by directing the mind to a single action. Contemplation is the next stage, when you are able to hold the image of an object or sound without allowing the mind to wander. You have achieved meditation when your mind becomes a continuous flow that is devoid of thought. When concentration becomes so intense that the continuous flow is absorbed, and when past, present and future merge, this is the state of actual meditation.

There are many ways to practice concentration. Perhaps the easiest way to begin is to focus on an object. Gaze at a work of art, a picture or statue, or if outdoors, at a flower, twig or a tree. Any object that is pleasing to your senses will do. Look steadily at the object for about three minutes. Don't let your gaze swerve or permit outside distractions to interfere.

Now close your eyes. Transfer your gaze to what the Yogis call the Third Eye, the area in the forehead between the eyebrows. Keep the image of the object in your mind as long as you can. Contemplate its color, shape and substance. The immediate response will be quite vivid, but the image will soon fade and begin to melt away. Try to hold onto it and bring it back. At first this will be difficult, but practice will make it easier to achieve. When you can no longer recall the image let go completely, emptying your mind of thought and impression. After awhile you may perceive lights, colored images, even metaphysical abstractions. Don't be afraid or try to repress them. Sink into these visions and let yourself float with them.

Concentration on the flame of a candle in the dim light or darkness is also effective. Close your eyes and hold the flicker of the flame in the Third Eye. Try to steady the flicker. When it recedes, order it back.

Another method of meditation is concentrating on sound: music, the song of a bird, even a fire siren. One of my favorite meditations is to concentrate on soft music: Bach, Haydn, Mozart, nothing too allegro. Rock music won't do. After awhile, you achieve awareness of every note and nuance. You learn to listen with every fiber of your body, becoming one with the sound.

TM claims that the Mantra used in meditation must be attuned to the student's individual vibrations. But a personal Mantra is not at all necessary for meditation. Any pleasing sound, word, aphorism or poem can be used. The effect results from persistent repetition at the same frequency. Choose a Mantra that feels comfortable to you. In the beginning stay with just one. Close your eyes, prepare your body through relaxation and breathing, and say the Mantra out loud to familiarize yourself with the sound. Now repeat it silently in a rhythm that is suitable for you, concentrating on the area of the Third Eye. If a thought wants to interfere, allow it to pass on. If it is a pressing one deal with it, then send it away and return to your Mantra.

You might want to experiment with concentrating on the breath. Relax your body, close your eyes and sit quietly. Breathe in through the nose on the count of one and exhale on two; inhale on three, exhale on four; and continue to the count of ten. Then go back to one and start over. Many people find this to be a very pleasant and effective practice of concentration. Experiment with different methods until you find one that works best for you. You may also enjoy guided meditation or guided imagery, in which an instructor or tape recording leads you through all the stages. This is a wonderful way to relax and recharge your energy.

When you start meditating you may feel self-conscious at first, even though you are completely alone. Remind yourself that it is essential for your well-being to become complete and whole. As you practice do not get discouraged. The beginning may be tedious but once you establish meditation as part of your daily routine, you will make progress each day, just as you have in your physical endeavors.

Do not begin with a preconceived goal in mind. Benefits will appear along the way. Meditation is not a planned journey. It is an exploration into the unknown for the discovery of the true self. The journey is exciting, because you can uncover a whole new realm of experiences that may exceed your most fervent hopes. You must allow it to happen. If you are not ready for change, accept yourself as you are and don't force alterations. You alone can judge what is right and comfortable for you.

Meditation As a Spiritual Experience

I believe meditation to be the true religion of mankind which has been overshadowed by organized religion, but can be recovered through diligent practice. Meditation leads one to the infinite, to union with the divine, no matter what name we call it. By searching the essence of ourselves, we seek the divine. Finding ourselves is to discover the Universal Spirit.

The God I speak of is in each of us. He does not reveal himself to a chosen few, but can be comprehended by all who seek him. Man chooses God. All religious scriptures try to teach human beings to look for inner peace through prayer and meditation. But man, it seems, has misinterpreted this to shift blame for his own shortcomings onto uncontrollable higher forces. Only when individuals find inner strength without reliance on outside forces can a better world evolve. Realizing that the answer to existence lies in the self, makes it possible to lead a meaningful life. When we stop blaming our failures on providence and learn to evaluate our faults honestly, we can liberate ourselves from fear and restore faith in the self.

Through meditation, we are able to free ourselves from preconceived concepts which we were taught because someone deemed them "good for us." As we open the Third Eye through meditation, we can penetrate the layers of falsehood and hypocrisy that have prevented us from knowing the truth about ourselves. Everyone is divine and can feel and experience their divinity by practicing inner reflection and meditation. Each of us can become strong and clear, so that we can lead ourselves through life with purpose and joy. And when the time comes, we can make a peaceful transition to the next life.

CHAPTER SEVEN

Spiritual Advancement

You Are Your Own Healer

We must open our minds and hearts to the realization that there is more to life than survival. We need to realize that we are in this life to learn and thereby create a better world. The practice of holistic thinking and living encourages us to overstep our limitations. Ridding ourselves of anxiety and fear through meditation will help us to be ready to take chances. An awakened mind is a curious mind, one that doesn't want to miss out on anything. If you are skeptical about healers, don't be dismayed. It is much better to be a skeptic and practice discrimination than to believe everything with no discernment. Even skepticism does not rule out an open mind.

When anyone mentioned faith, psychic or miracle healing, I used to be the biggest skeptic of all. I had made up my mind that all those who went to Lourdes, subsequently throwing away their crutches, were suffering from self-induced diseases. I was convinced that the "healings" produced by faith healers were the result of mass hysteria. I did not believe that any one person could have the mental powers to cure physical diseases in another individual. When I changed my mind, I discovered that fake healers do exist, but true ones are also prevalent. As I became interested in the subject, I read accounts of famous healers and met numerous others, availing myself of their treatments when necessary. I lost my skepticism but not my common sense. I always wanted proof, not someone's personal testimony. I met people who were merely attracting the gullible, but I also encountered people with true healing power. When they touched me, I often experienced a radiant heat that sent vibrations through my body. With other true healers, the results would speak for themselves.

There is nothing really miraculous about the power to

heal. Some are born with this special talent, others have developed the ability through practice and spiritual experiences. Many are unaware that they have this capacity, which I believe to be inherent in everyone. It is possible to train to become a healer. The universal life energy (or Prana) is present in all living things. A healing flow of energy permeates the atmosphere and can be tapped by everyone. There is also a rhythm-of-life energy that can be transmitted from one person to another and to animal and plant life as well.

I am a healer, but it took a long time for me to acknowledge my healing power. Although I studied with various practitioners, I lacked the confidence to apply what I learned. I discovered my own ability by chance when a student went into painful spasms in one of my Yoga classes. I intuitively put my hands on the afflicted area and the pain disappeared. I have seen scraped skin and open wounds disappear under my hands and I have applied emergency treatment whenever it is needed. But if someone with a chronic problem or disease needs my help, I do not only rely on my hands. In such cases, I apply and teach the holistic methods I know, or refer them to professional healers when indicated. I also accept and respect the reality that most dis-ease is self-induced and perpetuated for whatever reason, and do not wish to interfere.

There is almost no difference in psychic, spiritual or miracle healing. Essential to healing is the solid faith in oneself and in God, or whatever one wishes to call the highest energy. To receive acclaim is not the purpose of a healer. All true healers share one motivation: to alleviate suffering and to help mankind.

Even the most abject skeptic cannot maintain his doubts when confronted with irrevocable proof. The most amazing healer of our era was the American, Edgar Cayce, who died in 1945. Many who were suffering asked his advice and while he was in a trance their letters were read to him. He diagnosed nearly always accurately, and advised treatment for every conceivable illness, usually for people he had never seen. Cayce was known as the "Sleeping Prophet" and during his last years, as the "Miracle Man of Virginia Beach." He never went past the ninth grade in school. By profession, he was a photographer. In his everyday life, Cayce was a simple family man and a devout Christian. While in a trance he possessed an enormous knowledge of every branch of medicine, psychiatry, anatomy and chemistry. Many physicians turned to him for help with their unsolvable cases. His healing methods were unorthodox. He rarely advised surgery or chemical compounds, favoring herbal medicines, hydrotherapy, osteopathy, vitamin treatment and massage.

Cayce believed in the value of proper nutrition and is quoted as saying, "We are physically and mentally what we eat and think." His ideas were the forerunners to our present concepts of holistic health. The Edgar Cayce Foundation in Virginia Beach has well-catalogued records of more than 30,000 cases which he diagnosed in his lifetime. They are open to examination by any qualified individual. In the near future, more and more healers will want access to these facts.

Faith or spiritual healers are given more credence in other parts of the world, especially Great Britain where they have the endorsement of most of the medical profession. Many physicians who are unable to make progress with a case will refer the patient to a healer. Healers are permitted to assist physicians in hospitals and to administer last rites. In this country, interest has been aroused to the point where unorthodox healers sometimes lecture in medical schools and conduct workshops for doctors and students. Dolores Krieger, a professor of nursing at New York University, has successfully demonstrated that the "laying on of hands" by nurses and doctors affects changes in body temperatures and chemistry, producing remissions and cures. She has trained entire nursing staffs in various hospitals and her method is frequently endorsed by members of the medical profession.

Many writers and scientists are compiling testimonies of psychic healing that defy all scientific evidence. Psychic surgery is one example. Psychic surgeons in South America, Mexico, the Philippines and other areas operate with knives, hammers, chisels or their bare hands to remove tumors, cancers and ulcers. These methods sound far-fetched and many trained experts are trying to disprove them. One may choose to believe or to doubt those who have been cured. However, no incident has been recorded where someone has been harmed or injured by a psychic surgeon.

I place psychic and faith healers in the same category as physicians, chiropractors or other accredited healers. All are doing something for the patient and each is limited in his approach. But ultimately, while healers can change the symptoms of a disease, no one but the patient himself can reach the inner depths to change the process that produces the disease in the first place.

I have witnessed miraculous healings. People who have been confined to a wheelchair for many years got up and walked by themselves. The deaf heard sound, and I witnessed diseases disappear. But I feel these healings may be temporary if the cause of the disease has not been removed. A cancer, for instance, can only be subdued if the person is willing to locate the root of the growth and let it go. This root can be self-loathing, a deep resentment, or one of many hidden emotions. No cure can be lasting unless the patient changes his attitude toward sickness and health.

A good rapport between healer and patient is essential to effecting a cure. Faith in the healer, confidence in the doctor, is imperative to the success of the treatment. But faith in the self is really the ultimate answer. Every person has the ability to prevent disease and to cure it. Each of us has infinite power and if we choose, the ability to channel forces in the right direction. We may need assistance, but finally, we alone are our own true healers.

Psychics and Mediums

For most of my life I was petrified of the unknown and never had the slightest desire to explore it. I had been indoctrinated from earliest childhood with tales of ogres, monsters and bad witches who lie in wait for the unsuspecting. The popular children's literature that I read seemed to use monsters and witches to frighten children into following the orders of adults. The words psychic phenomena, occult and supernatural held ominous connotations for me. My strongest fear was of death. More than punishment for my sins, I feared the prospect of oblivion and loss of identity, for I was convinced that death was the total cessation of life.

When I began to listen to myself through meditation, I was gradually able to let go of fears that had paralyzed me throughout my life. The religious concepts of living and dying did not make sense to me. I decided to search for a satisfactory explanation for the purpose of existence.

In Yoga an adage states, "When the student is ready, the teacher will appear." My guru came to me, not as a dhoti-clad Hindu with a white beard, but as a corpulent, middle-aged British housewife. She is a world-famous clairvoyant and medium. I was in London attending a Yoga conference, and was at the time facing a severe domestic crisis. Friends had pushed me into seeking her advice. I was terrified of our first meeting and was determined to disbelieve whatever she said. She did, however, put me in touch with my departed husband and father, giving me the most detailed accounts of their characteristics. She made predictions about my future, which all came to pass. Her name is Doris Collins, and I call her "my psychic." Since we met, she has come to the United States several times to give readings, consultations and healings for my students and friends, and anyone else who needed help or guidance. She has enabled many people to overcome doubt, guilt and fear of death, uniting many with their loved ones in the spirit world.

I became aware of the spirit world which exists not above or below, but right here among us, in a different stratum or level of mind. Once I awakened to the existence of psychic interactions, I met many clairvoyants and spiritualists. I also encountered a vast group of "professional" seekers, who devote much of their time and money to exploring the occult. There are many gullible people who will take no action and make no decision without first consulting a psychic or their horoscope. But any reputable clairvoyant or astrologer will be the first to tell you that he or she is fallible. Predictions may be accurate only about eighty percent of the time. It is as sensible to consult a reputable psychic adviser in times of turmoil or indecision as it is to seek psychotherapeutic or other counseling. But no one has all the answers for you and it is imperative that you learn to trust yourself. Learn to rely on your own intuitive powers and apply them whenever possible. Realize that it is ultimately you who are in charge of your life.

The so-called occult sciences, like parapsychology and metaphysics, may not be acceptable to the conventional scientist who insists on logical facts, but these disciplines were an integral part of ancient civilizations. Astrology, for example, was the prevailing science among kings and statesmen throughout the Renaissance. Along with alchemy and the reading of the Tarot cards, it was considered an invaluable method for gaining knowledge. Original tenets of Judeo-Christian belief upheld esoteric practices as well. During the religious upheavals of the fifteenth century, however, the Catholic Church condemned the occult sciences as the devil's work. Practitioners were punished and put to death. Thousands of innocent people who allegedly practiced witchcraft were slaughtered in Europe and later in America.

In the nineteenth century, spiritualism and other healing

arts were revived in Britain. These arts also gained credence in the United States as part of the transcendentalists' movement. Various universities in the 1930s began research in psychic phenomena, including extrasensory perception and psycho-kinesis, the movement of physical objects by the mind without physical means. At Duke University, highly regarded studies were headed by Dr. J. B. Rhine. Rhine performed the difficult task of introducing psychic phenomena as a respectable sub-ject by renaming it parapsychology. The supernatural became the paranormal. Yet parapsychology or metaphysics is still a controversial subject in scientific circles. Although listed as an accredited course in many schools, no formal degree is issued in the field.

It is an open secret that our US government funds exten-sive research programs on psychic phenomena and the investi-gation of UFOs. Our researchers have to compete with those in the Soviet Union who are ahead of us in experiments with ESP, telepathy, psychic healing and psychokinesis. The Soviets are also very advanced in Kirlian photography, a technique that makes visible the auras, or fields of energy around every living being. One hopes, for the benefit of mankind, that the US and the USSR will eventually cooperate in psychic research, just as they have in the exploration of outer space. Great prog-ress in medicine and other sciences could be achieved if their studies were compared and combined.

Occultism, in various forms, has been actively practiced in the US in recent years, though it has operated primarily under-ground. Now it is merging into the mainstream. Astrological predictions have become a feature of most major publications and you can dial your horoscope by telephone. Hypnotists and psychics are employed by police departments to help solve crimes and find missing persons. Jeane Dixon, as President Roosevelt's personal psychic, became Washington's First Lady of Clairvoyance and we watched many of her predictions come true. She accurately predicted the assassination of President Kennedy. The media and general public opinion do not approve of fortune tellers — readers of palms, tarot, tea leaves and gazers into crystal balls — as well as they approve of prominent clair-voyants and parapsychologists. Yet the revelation in an obscure tearoom by a reader who charges $5.00 can be just as pro-found as a $100.00 reading by a top-notch psychic.

Fraudulence and fakery do exist in this field, as in other professions. Beware of the reader-adviser who distributes handbills or advertises in sleazy publications. For $2.00 per session, many of these people promise you love, health, fortune and the solution to each of your problems. Names like "Mrs. Emma" or "Sister Divine" are used and once you enter their premises, they may try to strip you of your resources by manipulating you with scare tactics or promises of greater wealth. Yet, even the con artists can be genuinely psychic. Most of them are West Indians or immigrants from Latin and South America, where psychic healers and seers are a part of native life. Gypsies, Indians (both Eastern and American) and other members of "primitive" societies are attuned to psychic phenomena, and psychic healing for them is a natural practice.

Most great inventions and discoveries result from flashes of insight or ESP. Among these are Einstein's theories and Edison's light bulb. The difference between an ordinary person and a genius is that the latter trusts his intuition. We all possess ESP. Everyone has insights, instinctive reactions and predictive impulses which, if acted upon, would usually prove to be right. How often do you say, "I was just going to say that," "You took the words right out of my mouth," or "I thought exactly what you were thinking"? We all experience precognitive dreams, bursts of enlightenment or déjà vu. Attempting a rational explanation, we term these events coincidence. We are programmed not to trust our intuition, out of fear of saying the wrong thing or making the incorrect decision. Children are innately psychic, but they are disbelieved, told not to make up such stories or assured that their imagination is running overboard. But having visions is not unusual. Being psychic or clairvoyant is a talent that is more pronounced in some than in others, like the gift for singing. It can, however, be developed by everyone. Basically it requires self-confidence, trust in one's intuitive power and belief in a higher consciousness. The first thought or impression that comes into one's mind is usually the right one. After being intellectualized the power of these flashes is lost.

You should exercise your psychic abilities, however, with discrimination. This is not a parlor game. Nor should consultation with a professional psychic or fortune teller be considered a frivolous pastime. It is wise to seek only those who have been recommended by someone you respect. Lots of pseudo-psychics proclaim their powers. Even if their motives are pure, they may suffer from delusions of grandeur, misleading others in turn. The same is true for spiritualists and mediums. People bereaved by the loss of loved ones and anxious to contact the spirit world are sometimes unable to exercise good judgment. They may fall prey to unethical or amateur practitioners. Be suspicious of those who need elaborate gimmicks or props to communicate with the spirit world.

Do not confuse spiritualism with spirituality, the seeking of higher consciousness. The two are not automatically linked. Since the beginning of time, there have been mediums or "sensitives" who act as intermediaries between the human world and the realm of spirits. They hear voices, either directly or in an altered state of consciousness which can be induced by prayer or meditation. Doris Collins starts each reading by thanking God for allowing her to be a channel. Edgar Cayce, who was a clairvoyant as well as a healer, communicated in a state of deep sleep. Then there are trance mediums who vacate their bodies, allowing another entity to speak directly through their physical form in a different voice or even a foreign tongue. This kind of channeling is the most celebrated form of psychic reading today. Examples of popular books on the subject are: *Argatha* by Meredith Young, the *Seth* books by Jane Roberts, the psychic communications by Ruth Montgomery and the *Ramtha* books channeled by J. Z. Knight. These authors and others have received messages from spirit guides who had important information to relate to the world.

Many in the spirit world are anxious to communicate with their loved ones on earth, to pass on important or sometimes innocuous messages to assure them that they are happy and well, and to encourage them not to grieve. Some in the spirit world need to heal earthly relationships or to be forgiven for their failures and wrongdoings in order to advance on their spiritual path. Others, who departed the earth without spiritual awareness, who were confused or mentally ill, died a sudden death or committed suicide may take longer to acknowledge their spiritual realm. But eventually, they too, will make every effort to contact the living.

A medium or go-between is not necessary for making contact with other dimensions. A variety of communication methods exist which anyone can employ, both believer and nonbeliever. It is possible to receive answers and messages from the spirit world via a pendulum, an Ouija board, the Chinese book of divination called the *I Ching,* automatic writing and meditation. Some serious seekers work in groups, particularly when using the Ouija board. An individual who is more psychic than the others can be chosen as the channel for messages and answers. Automatic writing needs no assistance. Anyone who is open can try this technique by lightly holding a pen or pencil poised over a piece of blank paper, or for the typist by placing the fingers gently on the keys, while in a meditative state. Written in this fashion, a number of books have been published containing material transmitted from outer forces. You can experiment with these methods; you may not always be successful, expecially when you begin, but one becomes adept with practice. Many lay people as well as metaphysical professionals condemn amateur attempts to communicate with the spirit world. They warn of discarnate or mischievous spirits who may want to confuse you. This may be true if you treat spirit communication as entertainment. But don't believe what you see in horror films! Spirit entities are not dangerous nor are they evil. Evil, like fear, is a state of mind. It only exists if you give it credence.

I knew I was communicating with the spirit world when my psychic knew the names and vital statistics of the people who were close to me. There was no way she could have had this information previously because we had never met before. I have a sound mind and I am sensible. I know that the pendulum I hold in my hand moves by itself. The pen writes with no help from me, and the planchette moves freely to spell out words on the Ouija board. (I also find it illogical to believe that we need to go through all the trouble of living on earth to be reduced to nothing but dust and ashes.)

Skeptics and dissenters will counter this with a series of rationalizations: pendulums (as well as dowsing rods) and planchettes emit radiation which activates nerve impulses that move the hand, automatic writing is a reflex set off by self-hypnosis, the subconscious mind has unknown powers which originate so-called messages from the spirit world. For every claim there is a contradiction. The doubter's view is as valid as the believer's. I can't blame anyone who doesn't share my enthusiasm. Until ten years ago, I thought the word spirit referred to alcohol!

Believers, especially enthusiasts, should be cautioned that communication with the spirit world, as with everything else, is not foolproof. Our concept of time, for instance, has no counterpart in the outer dimension because in this dimension time does not exist. An event predicted to occur "soon" may already have happened or may not happen for several years.

Any reference to time, therefore, should be taken with a grain of salt. Always employ common sense when contacting the spirit world.

Researchers and rationalists who are intent on proving that psychic phenomena are unrealistic and that life on earth is all there is, accomplish nothing more than the suppression of our spiritual nature. The so-called occult disciplines from the past have become the sciences of today. What were once considered miracles are now accepted as commonplace occurrences. These range from electricity and nuclear physics to the marvel of space travel. The existence of the spirit world will, in due time, be reaccepted as natural and will bear the stamp of scientific approval.

Death and Out-of-Body Experiences

Organized systems of belief—ancient Judeo-Christian, Asian and primitive religions of yesteryear and today— expound the concept of immortality. In many cultures, death is even celebrated as a joyous occasion in which a soul passes to a blissful afterlife. Such values and their ritual practices make it much easier to accept death for both the dying and the survivors. In our technological Western society we lack this confidence in our immortality. Our rational, three-dimensional minds are able to comprehend the intricacies of space travel, nuclear power, quantum physics and computer science, but in relation to ourselves, we can't seem to think beyond the physical body. Since we can't explain the function of the soul, we doubt its existence. We consider death as the finale of life, and we cloak it in secrecy. The dying are often shunned and robbed of their dignity. Too many of the elderly are put into hospitals so that they are out of the way and can die antiseptically.

Change, however, is on the way. We are being forced to acknowledge death as a normal part of life. Viewing it as a natural occurrence will erase its threatening aspects. Thanatology is the twentieth century science of death that deals with the physical process and the theoretical aspects of dying. One of the pioneers in the area of death and dying is Dr. Elizabeth Kubler-Ross, a physician and psychiatrist. Her book *Death and Dying* emphasizes the importance of open, honest communications with the dying. Her courageous efforts have caused a dramatic change in health professionals' attitude toward death. This change has led to the revival of hospices, a much more humane place than a hospital for accommodating the dying.

Kubler-Ross has also studied near-death experiences and investigated the esoteric aspects of afterlife. Her findings caused controversy among the conservative members of the medical profession, while stirring up interest among open-minded physicians and psychiatrists who have close contact with the dying.

Present research has resulted in a new wave of literature about near-death experiences. Written primarily by medical doctors, these books consist of comprehensive research as well as interviews with people pronounced clinically dead, who were later resuscitated. The compiled material is not derived from the vivid imagery of science fiction but from clinical accounts of people from all walks of life. Among the thousands interviewed no two stories are exactly alike, but all share striking similarities. For example, those who "die" in hospitals are often aware of the doctor pronouncing their death. They may hear a loud ringing, a buzzing or music before being pulled into a spiral, vacuum, or dark, seemingly endless tunnel. At the same time, they watch their past roll by like the rerun of a movie where every incident, deed, thought, dream and emotion of their life has been recorded.

When the noise stops or the tunnel ends, the supposed-dead may find himself floating on the ceiling of the hospital or operating room, trying to adjust to the novel situation. He is now in a body that cannot be seen. If he speaks, he cannot be heard. He is able to observe his lifeless body on the table being subjected to all kinds of resuscitation techniques, hooked into machines or pounded frantically on the chest by the doctors and nurses. Many people can recall the details of what was said, what everyone in the room looked like, and what instruments were being used. Then the individual sees beautiful colors or scenery and finds himself propelled toward an intense white light of indescribable beauty, which some identify as Christ or God. Departed relatives, friends, and sometimes religious figures come to meet the newly dead. Christians often relate that Jesus or Mary is there to greet them. Everyone encountered is loving and warm. The individual is overwhelmed by intense surges of love and peace and wants nothing more than to remain in the afterlife forever.

At this point he is advised gently by his loved ones that he must go back to earth. He is asked to return to finish what he set out to accomplish, or he is informed that others continue to need him. The person may be reluctant to take up the pain-ridden earthly existence again, but he does. Back in his earth body, he never forgets the death experience and is profoundly affected by it. His experience and new views make his life more meaningful. Not everyone experiences these events in the same sequence and not all of the clinically dead relate such pleasant or profound happenings. Some have no memory of the experience at all.

The body that replaces the physical one at the moment of death is the "astral" or "ethereal" body in current terminology. It was referred to as "Ka" in ancient Egypt, the "Shining Body" in the *Tibetan Book of the Dead,* and the "other body" in various Oriental texts. The psychic sees this phenomenon as an aura that surrounds the individual. In religious paintings it is the halo, and through Kirlian photography it appears as an energy field with spots of varying intensity. The ethereal body is perfect and whole when it detaches itself from the physical body. Those who had been diseased are suddenly healthy; amputees find they have legs and arms restored; the deaf can hear and the blind can see. Departed Yogis have been reported to assume their earthly forms looking years younger. According to the New Testament, those who saw Jesus when he returned to earth reported that he looked the same as before the crucifixion.

Astral projection and out-of-body experiences are not confined to the moment of death. Some people can temporarily break away from the physical plane. When they return, they recount their travels, telling of experiences which are outside of our everyday concepts of time and place. The out-of-body experience may take place spontaneously, in sleep, at the brink of sleep, during meditation or during other altered states of consciousness. It can also be induced by hypnotism, autosuggestion or in laboratory experiments with polygraphs and other apparatus.

Those who tell of astral projection say that body consciousness and the preconception of "I" is transcended, but no two experiences are alike. Some observe their physical form sitting on a chair or couch listening to a family discussion while their astral body floats above the scene. Others visit the home of relatives, friends or strangers. Some can travel at the speed of light to distant cities and countries, even other planets. Sometimes they are seen by witnesses who report apprehending Doppelgangers or doubles. This is an experience that can occur once in a lifetime, or frequently. Usually it is joyful and thrilling, promoting greater awareness in one's life.

Explanations of this phenomenon differ. The skeptic refers to it as dreaming or coincidence. Psychiatrists may label it hysteria, hallucination or autoerotic longing. Others, physicists, neurologists and psychoanalysts like Carl Jung, have joined with parapsychologists and metaphysicists to research and document the ever-increasing evidence of out-of-body experience.

Some who observe the dying at the actual moment of death see the soul leave the body in the form of a white light or cloud. Photographic experiments will, in time, make this phenomenon visible. Many who wait at a death bed see the facial expression of the dying change from pain and fear into a peaceful smile. Others report a similarity in final words, such as "Here is John," referring to a loved one who passed away previously. Some pass this off as hallucination, but it is proof to the believer that no one dies alone. Whether a person dies in bed or in the desert, he will be met by a spirit guide, many times by the same one who was at his side at the moment of birth. Everyone is assisted when making the transition between planes, from the physical body to the astral body.

Reincarnation and Karma

Reincarnation and karma used to be, to me, additional aspects of Yoga that were interesting but not relevant to Western thought. The incarnations of Vishnu, Siva and Krishna seemed to be nothing but whimsical folklore. I maintained that the prospect of reincarnation provided an excuse for the masses of India to cop out in this lifetime, because they felt they could always do better the next time around. I felt that the belief in karmic retribution perpetuated the caste system and allowed cows and other creatures that spread disease to roam freely over India. I felt that the recall of past-life experiences could be explained by genetic memory or dreams or subconscious childhood impressions. I was fond of pointing out that without eye witness accounts, there is no scientific evidence of reincarnation. I also never found any references to the afterlife in Western culture. Even if I had confronted a karmic experience, I would have ignored such information because of my lack of awareness and my disbelief. Like most of us, I knew only what I had been programmed to know by the society of my generation.

I was not a religious person and I shuddered at the prospect of the destruction of my body. I believed that no one had ever returned from the grave. Only when I met "my psychic" did I begin to see the light. The concept of reincarnation, the rebirth of one's soul into a new body, made sense for the first time and provided me with a reasonable explanation for the phenomena of death and the unequal opportunities that are present for the living. I began to read accounts of people who, through hypnosis or the supervised administration of hallucinogens, were able to recall past lives, stating details that were subsequently documented. Great thinkers like Plato, Socrates, Voltaire, Emerson and Thoreau all believed in reincarnation, as did practical men like Ben Franklin, Mark Twain, Arthur Conan Doyle, Henry Ford and Edgar Mitchell, the American astronaut. As I started to believe in an afterlife, I found more and more people who shared my beliefs. I came to realize that whatever happened to me in this life is neither chance, coincidence, disposition nor inheritance. My parents, husband, children, relatives, friends and acquaintances all came into my life for a reason.

One of the most forceful arguments of skeptics is that no one remembers their past lives in the present. But no one remembers the events of babyhood either! You would also draw a blank if you were asked what you did on August 7, five years ago. Past lives can be recalled through hypnosis or regression techniques, and are often verified by authenticated research. Psychiatrists and psychologists have attested that the recall of past lives can help in the treatment of deep-seated psychological problems, or offer an explanation for erratic behavior.

Reincarnation can be seen as a cycle within the evolutionary process of existence. Everything in our world follows a cyclic order: summer follows winter, day follows night. All things in nature — plants, trees, oceans, land masses — are continually recycled. Reincarnation can be viewed as a recycling technique through which the immortal self discovers the purpose and godliness of existence. When we accept reincarnation, we see life as a pilgrimage toward truth and perfection which leads to a magnificent outcome. We realize that nothing is futile or without significance and lasting value. Everything is a learning experience.

Each incarnation is an opportunity for greater development that takes us nearer to the goal of perfection. Grief, agony and guilt can be emotions of the past. All we need to acknowledge is that we made mistakes or errors of judgment. No one else can judge or punish us. We, ourselves, are the ones to evaluate this life or previous lives and correct them. It is only necessary to become aware of each error and to recognize its adverse effect on ourselves and others. We learn to view every negative action of our past as a learning process that moves us toward greater understanding, but we also see the need to rectify our mistakes, and are anxious to undo any hurt inflicted on ourselves or on others.

Karma is the Hindu and Buddhist cosmic principle of universal law. It is a Sanskrit word that means total responsibility for all actions. It is the explanation and justification of good or bad fortune during one's life. It can be interpreted as action and reaction, cause and effect. In the Bible, karma is reflected in the adage, "As ye sow, so shall ye reap." Every word, idea and action during a lifetime produces either positive or negative effects. The ensuing results must be balanced out by experience in another lifetime. This doctrine does not lend itself to the Hindu's resignation, since the present life is not meant for procrastination, but for progress and growth. Each time on earth, in whatever circumstance or body we choose, we have the chance and free will to work out our karma, amending the consequences of our past lives. Karma is not doled out, it is self-induced. As individuals we do not always accomplish what we hoped to in one lifetime. But we never waste a life or get a failing mark, and there is always another chance.

Everyone has the ability to end his karmic debt once and for all. Man possesses free will on earth and can change his destiny if he so chooses. You do not need to accept traits in yourself that don't please you. For example, you don't need to say, "I am stubborn because I am a Taurus," or "I am an Aries, that is why I am so impatient." Instead, as an indication of your spiritual growth, you might say: "I used to be a Gemini, two people, always divided. But now I have unified myself." God created man, but man is the co-creator. He can overcome his karmic circumstances and rise above them. A child raised in ignorance and poverty can adjust mentally as well as physically to function beautifully in spite of his handicaps. Helen Keller is a perfect example. Born deaf and blind, she changed the course of her life and rose triumphantly as an inspiration for the whole world. Karmically speaking, no one takes on more than can be handled in one lifetime. Those who seem to be victims of all the miseries in the world have an ability to endure them. Individual and collective guilts do not have to be carried over into another life. Awareness of a mistake — recognition of a wrong — can correct it in an instant.

Karmic action takes on an enriched meaning and leads to more definite results once the principle of karma is understood and applied. Yet it is subject to much misinterpretation. Ironically, this is particularly true in India where karmic awareness is high. The Bhagavad Gita states that the release from future karma lies in impersonal detachment from action. The Eastern Indian takes this idea literally, displaying indifference, even callousness toward those who suffer. He takes it for granted that all unfortunates are atoning for misdeeds and should be left to their misery. Those in the West who believe in karmic law do not apply this philosophy. Westerners most often follow the moral principles of Judeo-Christian religions that call for compassion and brotherly love.

We are not personally responsible for the suffering of others. We did not single-handedly create world starvation. We do not have to be devastated by pity and guilt, but we certainly cannot be indifferent. All of us are connected in a universal sense, and for that reason, do carry moral obligations to one another. Compassion is a positive human emotion. By offering love and hope, we may influence someone else to change his karma, diminishing our own debt at the same time.

Schopenhauer believed the Western world to be unique in its incredible delusion that man was created out of nothing, that his present birth is the first entrance into life. Voltaire said that it should be no more surprising to be born twice than to be born once. Paul Brunton, an expert on Oriental philosophy, is convinced that the survival of Western civilization depends on the restoration of karmic ideas in the thinking of the masses. The knowledge of karma and reincarnation is a holistic as well as common sense attitude toward life. It is a positive approach to human existence, encouraging maturity along with the certainty of finding meaning and purpose in everyday living.

We all have to achieve cosmic consciousness to save our planet. We can't just hope that things will improve, that problems will solve themselves. We created war and the destruction of the planet. We can create peace and heal the earth. We can't count on a few sages who pray for salvation to bring about world peace nor can we wait for a Messiah to save mankind. Each of us can contribute by making peace a way of life in our homes and in our work. But the peace must start within each of us.

About the Author

Ina Marx is the author of *Yoga and Common Sense,* published by Bobbs-Merrill and translated into three languages. It first appeared as a hardcover edition in 1970, and was completely revised for publication in 1977. Ina has lectured widely; she has appeared on radio and television and has been featured in magazine and newspaper articles. As founder and director of the Yoga for Long Island institute in New York, she has taught Hatha-Yoga, meditation, relaxation, and stress control for over twenty years. She is considered to be an authority on Yoga and Eastern philosophies along with all phases of holistic health. Ina practices holistic principles, including consciousness raising, spiritual awareness, healing techniques and mind therapies. Currently, she is engaged as a holistic counselor and conducts workshops on transformation and growth.

You can write to her at any time for personal advice or just to ask questions. She is also available for lectures and demonstrations, and conducts workshops in various areas of California.

Ina Marx
P.O. Box 91
Tiburon, California 94920